WHEN YOUR LOVED ONE HAS ALZHEIMER'S

WHEN YOUR LOVED ONE HAS *Alzheimer's*

A CAREGIVER'S GUIDE

DAVID L. CARROLL

BASED ON METHODS DEVELOPED BY

THE BROOKDALE CENTER ON AGING

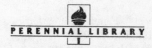

PERENNIAL LIBRARY

Harper & Row, Publishers, New York

Grand Rapids, Philadelphia, St. Louis, San Francisco
London, Singapore, Sydney, Tokyo, Toronto

The Library of Congress has catalogued the hardcover edition as follows:

Carroll, David.
When your loved one has alzheimer's.

Includes index.
1. Alzheimer's disease—Patients—Family relationships.
2. Married people. I. Carroll, David, 1942-
II. Brookdale Center on Aging (Hunter College)
RC523.W49 1989   618.97'683   88-45569
ISBN 0-06-015887-5

ISBN 0-06-091667-2 (pbk.)

90 91 92 93 94 FG 10 9 8 7 6 5 4 3 2 1

Contents

Acknowledgments

I would like to take this opportunity to thank the following people and acknowledge their help: Dr. David Kamlet, for several hours of sympathetic, to-the-point interview time; Dr. Ken Davis, for his incisive presentation of the current Alzheimer's picture; Dr. Nancy Foldi, clinical psychologist at Mount Sinai Hospital, for her intelligent insights; Dr. Lynne Clark, for providing me with some of the most substantial material in this book; Dr. Virginia Barrett, for her brilliant perceptions and giving nature; Clauda Girling-Zanger, for her interest; Richard Anderson, for his efforts and legal input; Jeannette Richardson, for all the generous information, and for just being herself; Honey Zimmer, for help getting started; Arlene McCormick, for help finishing up; Dr. Rick Moody, for getting the ball rolling and for stopping the buck; Dr. Rose Dubrof, for her warm and loving support; Dr. Robert Barrett, one of the very best; Rea Khan, for introducing me to many courageous people, and for her compassion; Dr. Gertrude Steinberg, for her time and advice; Dr. Sharon Shaw, for valuable insights; Dr. Judah Ronch, one of the most enlightened professionals currently working in the field today; John Jaeger, for showing me the Alzheimer's Disease and Related Disorders Association (ADRDA) from the inside; Dr. Ben Lessiman, for giving more time than he had; Dr. Della Dorman and Dr. John Dorman, neurologists par excellence. Special thanks to Marilyn Howard at Brookdale, without whose help this book would be half. And to caregivers too numerous to name—so many thanks.

Introduction

This is a book on Alzheimer's disease written expressly for caregivers. Several works dealing with the management of this difficult disease have been published over the past few years, and most of them are substantial presentations, filled with sympathetic, hands-on information. A majority of these offerings, however, suffer from a kind of blind spot, a failure to fully inform and stand behind the "second victim" of Alzheimer's disease, the psychic victim, the person who must trail behind the patient and pick up the pieces.

This person is, of course, the caregiver—you. Placed in a guardianship position for which you were probably never trained and about which you certainly have mixed emotions, you may suddenly find yourself cast in a number of new and unfamiliar roles—parent, nurse, social director, punching bag, and savior, to name just a few—all for the exclusive purpose of aiding a loved one stricken by the relentless disorder we call Alzheimer's. Perhaps you are the spouse of such a person; perhaps the child, the close friend, the companion, the grandchild, or some other caring relative. Whatever your relationship, this book is for your use and your benefit. It is written to help you cope better, to serve the patient better, and to ensure your survival in the process.

The information and techniques you will find in these pages are designed to be used on several levels, some practical, some psychological, a few spiritual. Read the text through and mark off the sections you find particularly applicable. Then turn to these sections when the need arises. Use this book as a resource and reference, as a how-to manual, as a companion to guide you through difficult times. Let it complement your work with the physician and other health care personnel. Let it arm you for the strenuous months ahead. The techniques and advice featured here have given hope and support to thousands of people through the years. They can help you too.

Meet the Brookdale Center on Aging

All material offered in this book is based on information provided by a coterie of professional health care workers who in one way or another are affiliated with the Brookdale Center on Aging. One of the largest and most active geriatric facilities in the United States, the Brookdale Center is located in New York City adjacent to Bellevue Hospital in downtown Manhattan. It is affiliated with New York's Hunter College and is involved in a wide range of social as well as medical issues, almost all of them related to the process of human aging.

A good part of the Brookdale Center's work focuses on the problems of Alzheimer's and related dementias, both at the research level and on a practical, day-to-day basis. Brookdale discovered early in the game that it is the relatives of Alzheimer's sufferers who usually end up serving as the primary caregivers and who are forced to shoulder the physical, financial, and emotional responsibilities that attend this complex ailment. The staff of Brookdale therefore decided that they owed it to these dedicated people to provide them with a reference work describing the practical lessons Brookdale's staff and associates have learned concerning the care of Alzheimer's patients, and revealing the many obvious and not-so-obvious methods they have developed through the years to make home care more efficient.

Thus Brookdale put together a preliminary outline based on their work with elderly patients and then contacted the author. After several meetings with Brookdale's staff and with the publishers, Harper & Row, the author spent more than a year in the field speaking directly with a wide range of patients, caregivers, and health care professionals, gathering important Alzheimer's-related materials. Most of these professionals were affiliated with the Brookdale Center, and all of them were sympathetic to Brookdale's philosophy: "Treat the patient as well as the disease; treat the caregiver as well as the patient."

This group of professionals included M.D.'s, social workers, psychologists, medical researchers, psychiatrists, nurses, rehab personnel, heads of self-help organizations, and many more, all of whom willingly offered their time and knowledge to make this book definitive.

The instructions offered in this program, therefore, are based on state-of-the-art scientific work accomplished by scores of medical researchers and, perhaps more important for our purposes, on years of hands-on experience in the field of geriatric home care by Brookdale's professionals. Followed on a regular basis, this information will show you how to deal with a variety of logistic problems for both patient and caregiver. It will likewise: (1) describe new methods for successful day-to-day management of home-bound Alzheimer's patients; (2) address the difficult emotional decisions that will have to be made at every turn of the way; (3) provide guidance in financial and logistical matters; and (4) tell caregivers how, in the face of the many responsibilities which beset them, to best look after their own physical and emotional needs in the process.

The author and the many health care professionals who have contributed to this book unanimously consider you, the caregiver in an Alzheimer's situation, to be the true unsung hero of our story. Demented persons tend to look hale and hearty in the early days of their disease, unlike victims of many other terminal ailments. When a relative at home is visibly withering away from cancer or a heart problem, it is not difficult for friends and neighbors to sympathize and to offer their full-fledged help. But when the so-called patient looks and acts almost the same as before, compassion comes more grudgingly, if at all. Sometimes even the Alzheimer's caregiver becomes the butt of well-meaning but basically critical advice. "But your husband looks so healthy!" is a common phrase. "You should be grateful." Or, "Well, at least your Laura is up and about at home. Poor Ruth, what with that arthritis and diabetes—now *there's* a problem."

Despite the fact that the ailing person seems fine to the misted-over eyes of the world, however, professionals who work in the field of demential diseases know all about the quiet struggles that go on behind closed doors. They know about the patient's temper tantrums, the incontinence pads, the embarrassing scenes in restaurants and banks. They have witnessed the hands that can no longer grip a fork and the brains that can no longer remember how to count to ten. Most of all, they know the real meaning of the decision caregivers have come to, to keep their ailing loved ones at home for the time being, to provide them with hour-by-hour nursing care, even though this decision means, in effect, giving up their own private lives.

Health care professionals in this field have witnessed all these events, and they know what you are going through. Those that have participated in this book thus unite in their hope that what you read in these pages will give you confidence in the midst of difficulty and that the practical assistance you gain here will help to lighten your very heavy load.

PART I
UNDERSTANDING
ALZHEIMER'S DISEASE

1

Getting to Know the Enemy: Understanding Alzheimer's Disease

"But she's acting so strangely all of a sudden . . ."

One day when Margaret C. was sixty-eight years old, she started behaving strangely. Living in a large condominium apartment in a relatively affluent section of Lansing, Michigan, Margaret shared this opulent space with her divorced daughter, Ann, and her daughter's six-year-old son, Jimmy. Margaret's husband had died of a heart attack two years earlier, and though grief-stricken at the loss, she continued to work at her job as a legal secretary, more to keep her mind off her sadness than to make a living (Margaret's husband had left her a healthy inheritance).

In most ways and to most people, Margaret seemed a gentle, well-adjusted woman, much given to propriety and to life's fixed daily routines. It thus seemed strange to her daughter when Margaret started leaving for work on certain days through the back door rather than the front. Ann didn't think much about this incongruous change until one day she noticed her mother pack Jimmy's lunch, hand it to him, then pack it again a few minutes later. Odd.

Margaret's dressing habits also took a curious turn. Sometimes she wore shoes that didn't match. Sometimes her color combinations were, quite atypically, tasteless and occasionally even ludicrous. Margaret would forget to button her blouse all the way down. She would leave her apartment on a stormy day without a raincoat, then resent being told about it. She would grope for a simple word to express a simple idea or occasionally entirely lose track of what she was saying in the middle of a sentence. She became uncharacteristically cranky when the grapefruit didn't slice properly. She swore at the maid.

For Ann the most confusing part of this new scenario was that there really was no particular pattern to any of these deviations and lapses. Sometimes her mother dressed normally. Sometimes she left through the front door. But sometimes she did things that she had simply never done before. This worried Ann. She decided to talk to her mother.

Though they had gone through some rocky times together when Ann was first married, Margaret and her daughter had grown closer since the divorce and by now had achieved a more or less honest exchange of feelings. Yet when Ann let her mother know what was on her mind, Margaret not only professed unawareness of what Ann was talking about but became immediately offended. In fact, Margaret made it seem as if *Ann* were the strange one, the "sick one," for worrying her head about such picayune things.

So Ann sloughed it off. But the mistakes and the lapses kept coming, and they became progressively worse—not all at once, but over weeks and months. Eventually it became clear to Ann, her friends, even the neighbors and the local clerks and shopkeepers that something was truly amiss. Margaret was definitely changing, they all agreed, and not in a positive way.

It finally took the testimony of three of Margaret's closest friends plus the urgings of her boss at the law firm (he had noticed that Margaret was forgetting to inform him about appointments and was misplacing important documents) to go to a physician. Reluctantly, nervously, angrily, Margaret complied.

After a thorough checkup at a medical clinic, a complete neurological examination that included an hour of psychological testing, and more than a month of waiting for the results, the doctor called Ann and Margaret to a meeting in her office. Though she could not be one hundred percent certain, the doctor explained—a totally positive diagnosis can be arrived at only by autopsy or by a brain biopsy—it seemed reasonably clear to her from the tests and examination that Margaret was suffering from a variety of dementia. The dementia was, the doctor said, in all probability Alzheimer's disease.

What Is Alzheimer's Disease?

After Margaret's diagnosis was delivered and pondered over, Ann requested a second, private meeting with the doctor. Just what was

Alzheimer's disease? She wanted to know. How could the doctor be certain of her diagnosis? What precisely were the symptoms? How fast would the disease develop? What would it do to her mother? Was it fatal? What did it all mean?

Alzheimer's disease, the doctor explained, or AD as it is often called, is a form of *dementia*, a global neurological impairment characterized by slowly progressive and irreversible deterioration of the cognitive functions—speech, abstract thought, emotion, memory—and hence of the ability to take care of oneself, to identify time and place, to relate socially to others, to think and speak and act in a clear and reasonable way.

AD can be biologically characterized, the doctor added, by actual atrophy of the cortical regions of the brain (the cortex is the outer, gray layers of the cerebral lobes) and behaviorally by a set of dramatic and deviant alterations in the patient's social personality.

To understand what all this means, the doctor explained, it is necessary to focus on the term *dementia*. This is an emotionally charged word that AD caregivers will hear again and again. The term itself derives from the Latin *de*, meaning "from," and *mentis*, meaning "mind." Contrary to some people's understanding, it does not refer to a particular disease but encompasses a variety of disorders, of which Alzheimer's is one of the most common.

Dementias can be triggered by a number of unrelated situations and not necessarily by a single cause. Take some typical examples. In one case a patient may suffer dementia due to a series of small, indetectable strokes. In another the side effects of medications may be the cause. In a third a haymaker punch that pounds a person's brain a little too hard against the back of the skull is to blame (the typical punch-drunk boxer is often suffering from a kind of dementia).

Sometimes dementias are temporary and reversible. Sometimes they are not. AD is not. Whatever the case may be, when presented with a possible case, the physician's first task is to determine whether the disorder at hand actually *is* dementia—there are many dementia look-alikes, as we will see—and then to take the appropriate steps.

Unfortunately, an AD diagnosis is further complicated by the fact that the symptoms of different dementias tend to look more or less alike from the outside, even though the causes behind them may be quite different. Therefore, the first thing a doctor must do after having eliminated all dementia look-alikes from the diagnostic picture is to establish the cause of this particular dementia, then determine whether it is reversible or irreversible, progressive or nonprogressive, temporary or permanent.

What are the different causes of dementias that must be ruled out before it can be said that the disorder is actually AD? Here is a comprehensive though far from definitive list:

- Multi-infarct dementia (MID) (stroke damage)
- Parkinson's disease
- Huntington's disease
- Spinocerebellar degeneration
- Amyotrophic lateral sclerosis ("Lou Gehrig's disease")
- Rare nerve diseases: kuru, Pick's disease, Wilson's disease, Creutzfeldt-Jakob disease

These represent the main *irreversible* forms. Though none on the list is currently curable, the symptoms of certain ailments, such as Parkinson's disease, can in many cases be kept under control with medication.

The following are the most common causes of potentially reversible dementias:

- Hypothyroidism and hyperthyroidism
- Renal failure
- Neurosyphilis
- Dehydration
- Reactions to medication
- Brain tumor
- Addison's disease
- Head trauma (with subdural hematoma)
- Hyperglycemia
- Malnutrition
- Liver disease
- Lupus erythematosus
- Hypopituitarism
- Viral infections
- Vitamin B_{12} or thiamine deficiency
- Chemical or environmental poisoning
- Congestive heart failure
- Lack of electrolyte balance
- Acid-base disturbance
- Anesthesia
- Chronic alcoholism

Counted up, physicians estimate that more than sixty disorders can produce dementia.

Ann could now understand why her mother's symptoms called for such a thorough examination and why so many hours of testing are required before a clinical determination of Alzheimer's can be suggested.

Inside the Brain of an Alzheimer's Patient

Before finding out how physicians and, to a limited extent, caregivers can help recognize dementia and its look-alikes, it will be helpful to gain a working knowledge of the physical events that actually occur in the brain of an AD sufferer.

As you may already know, in 1906 a German scientist named Dr. Alois Alzheimer discovered Alzheimer's disease to be a form of dementia. As fate would have it, he based his findings on samples of brain tissue taken from a woman who died of the disease, quite uncharacteristically, at age fifty-five. And so for some years after his discovery, Alzheimer's disease was assumed to affect only middle-aged patients. Those older men and women who did happen to exhibit AD-like behavior were accordingly dismissed as being "a little dotty" and were relegated to the rocking chair and attic.

It was not until the late 1950s that doctors began to understand that what had been described, somewhat tongue-in-cheek perhaps, as "mental decrepitude" was, in certain cases, more than just the result of normal aging. They now realized that senility was an actual disease, one that required clinical treatment plus a good deal of specialized care. In fact, over the past quarter century, physicians have come to find out that Alzheimer's disease afflicts not just a tiny slice of the geriatric population but almost one million Americans a year and that it has now become the fourth largest contributive cause of death in the United States.

These are formidable statistics, made all the more vivid by the fact that they were recognized only recently and that so many people still remain unaware of the Alzheimer's menace. Alzheimer's disease and related dementias are with us everywhere, a kind of "silent epidemic," as one writer described it, and they thus concern every person approaching old age. For example, if you are sixty-five years of age at the present time, you have approximately a ten percent probability of developing Alzheimer's disease within the next year. A decade and a half later your odds will go up to forty percent. And if you continue into your eighties, the time will come when your chances of succumbing to complications caused by Alzheimer's disease will be fifty percent. It's serious business.

What, then, actually happens physiologically to the demented patient to produce this fatal debilitation? If we take a sample of our friend Margaret's brain cells and study them microscopically, what will we find?

Initially, probably nothing, until we focus in on two specific areas. The first is the outer mantle—the cortex—of the frontal and temporal cerebral lobes. The second is the hippocampus, a small, gracefully curved elevation (its name is derived from the Greek word for "seahorse," which it vaguely resembles) located directly below the cerebral cortex and responsible, in part, for short-term memory.

If we perform a biopsy on these two sections and remove discrete samples for analysis, we will observe three irregularities which are not found to any great extent in normal brain matter. These irregularities go by the names of *neurofibrillary tangles*, *neuritic plaques*, and *granulo-vacuolar degeneration*.

Neurofibrillary Tangles.   Since a picture is worth a dozen paragraphs, glance at the drawings in Figure 1.1. Picture A depicts a normal brain cell. It is known as a *neuron*. Interestingly enough, it is shaped something like a tree shed of its leaves. At the base of this tree is the cell's nucleus, and growing out of it is a "trunk" with many "branches." This trunk is the *axon*, and the branches are known as *dendrites*. Leaping from neuron to neuron over tiny gaps called *synapses*, coded impulses travel along the length of these innumerable connections at speeds of several hundred miles an hour. By means of an electrochemical process that is only partially understood at this time, their movements ultimately produce the endless numbers of mental transmissions we know as thought, reason, memory, emotion, and physiological functioning.

Now picture B: Notice that the shape of the neuron has changed here, in an ominous way. A number of the dendrites are missing, and worse, the nucleus is filled with a mass of intertwined protein filaments that in certain ways resemble steel wool. These masses are the *neurofibrillary tangles*.

Almost everyone among the elderly population will have a few of these helix-shaped bundles in their gray matter. They are a normal indicator of advancing age. But in the brains of Alzheimer's sufferers they begin to appear in great profusion, not only in the cell nucleus but near the axons and dendrites as well. These tangles are an indication that the cell is disintegrating. Their presence, especially in the temporal and frontal lobes and in the hippocampus, provides a strong indication of Alzheimer's disease.

Figure 1.1.   Stages of neuron degeneration

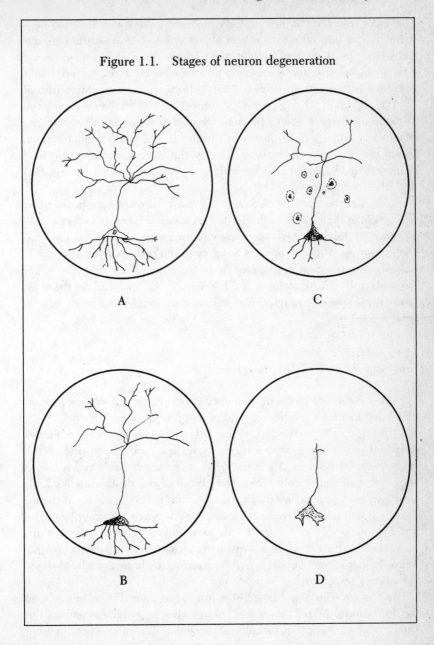

Senile Neuritic Plaques.   Study picture C. Near the decaying den-drites notice several small, round objects, the *senile neuritic plaques.* These masses of amyloid protein material are composed of residues left over from healthy nerve endings, now broken off and decayed. Their presence in the cell provides further indication of deterioration caused by AD, especially when a biopsy (or autopsy) places them in the company of neurofibrillary tangles. In fact, when a massive number of these plaques and tangles are observed lurking in the frontal and temporal lobes and in the hippocampus, this is the most persuasive piece of diagnostic evidence we have for making a positive clinical determination of Alzheimer's disease.

Granulovacuolar Degeneration.   A third danger sign appears when tiny granular materials and fluid-filled vacuoles are seen crowding inside the body of the nerve cell, specifically in the pyramid-shaped cells of the hippocampus. This condition, known as *granulovacuolar degeneration,* can only be observed in biopsied brain tissue and then only after it has been carefully sliced, stained, and microscopically analyzed. In the com-pany of plaques and tangles, it is yet another sign of neuron deteriora-tion.

Stages of Brain Cell Degeneration

What is the fate of the neuron once it begins the unforgiving process of decay? Picture D shows the end of its grim journey.

Here the cell, having lost its dendrites and nucleus, withers in ear-nest and soon disintegrates entirely, vanishing forever into the body's waste disposal systems. The deterioration of a single brain cell is incon-sequential, of course, but when this plague of cell deaths repeats itself over and over in concentrated sections of the brain, whole areas die en masse. Eventually the consequences of this wastage become plain. The surface topography of the cortex grows visibly altered and displays un-characteristic pitting, wide fissures, crags, and an overall loss of weight. With the depletion of enough nerve material, the brain actually shrinks, sometimes by as much as ten percent.

The more cells the AD sufferer loses, the more his or her mental faculties erode. After years of such neural atrophy, vital functions of the thinking apparatus are drastically diminished, and some functions have disappeared entirely, leaving severely reduced cognitive and motor skills. Persons who were once witty, cordial, and quick on their feet are now reduced to the status of deranged children—or worse. Exactly what triggers this inexorable process of degeneration we do not yet know.

When to Bring Your Loved One to the Doctor

As you will recall, the abrupt change in behavior patterns that Margaret demonstrated at home and in her office quickly became evident to just about everyone around her. But are early symptoms of dementia always so easy to catalog and so well defined?

No, not always, and neither are there any hard-and-fast diagnostic rules that families can apply to determine whether an oldster's erratic behavior really warrants a costly trip to the doctor. The one sure-fire method of identifying AD, as mentioned earlier, can be done only after the fact with a brain autopsy. Until then no diagnosis will ever be one hundred percent accurate. The American Psychiatric Association once even recommended that doctors not use the term "Alzheimer's disease" at all but that they opt for the more conservative label "primary degenerative dementia."

At the same time, families surely need some set of general guidelines for determining whether an elderly relative is showing signs of AD or is simply getting older. These guidelines do exist, as we shall see. But happily, in probably a majority of cases, the personality alterations that families fret over in elderly relatives are not Alzheimer's disease at all but a wide range of possible physical and emotional problems, many of which are reversible.

Sometimes, for instance, disorientation or memory loss may be caused by disguised alcohol abuse (it is a little-known fact that the largest segment of the alcoholic population in the United States is made up of widows over the age of sixty-five). Infections occasionally produce dementialike personality alterations, as do reactions to medications. Often the culprit is simply the normal aging process.

How, then, can you differentiate these conditions one from the other? And when do you know for certain that the changes are serious enough to seek health care? Let's have a look at both questions up close.

Is It Really a Problem?

The older a person gets, the more likely a family is to anticipate, unconsciously perhaps, that at any moment the elderly one will come down with a slow, terrible, killing disease. Observe some examples:

Mom's breathing is dreadfully labored now after climbing just a few stairs. Isn't Grandma's face turning red for no particular reason when she talks? Why has Dad forgotten to tie his shoes for the hundredth time? Such unnerving observations cause family members to stab nervously at the panic button: Mom's got lung cancer; Grandmother's suffered a stroke; Dad has Alzheimer's disease. These terrors, fortunately, soon prove to be inaccurate as the weeks and months go by. Nothing is really wrong with these persons, it turns out. They are simply getting older.

Of all the alarming symptoms that elderly persons may demonstrate, memory loss is the most noticeable. Old people simply forget more things than they used to, and they do it in a more obvious way. They will leave the water running in the sink or neglect to close the front door. They may repeat themselves several times in the same conversation. Or you'll hear the same stories related three times a day. They may forget the name of the dog, the letter carrier, or a grandchild. For a moment they may even forget *your* name.

None of these mental slips are necessarily cause for worry, and families would be well advised in instances of forgetfulness to opt for the benefit of the doubt. The rule of thumb is not to worry (1) if an older person's memory lapses and violations of common sense are minor and temporary, (2) if they do not become progressively worse in a relatively short period of time, (3) if they are not bizarre or out of character, and (4) if they seem to be logical exaggerations of the person's regular personality. They are most likely caused by Father Time. He will visit all of us sooner or later.

When to Get Worried

There's a magic line that separates the ordinary foibles of old age from the true symptoms of disease. In many cases, perhaps in most, you will have little trouble identifying when that line has been crossed— especially if you know what you're looking for.

To begin, you have probably already been told that memory impairment is the first danger signal in Alzheimer's disease. This advice, if not entirely incorrect, is incomplete. Become concerned with memory loss only when it represents *unusual* or *uncharacteristic* degrees of forgetting. Become more concerned when you observe atypical lapses into disorientation and/or disorganization on the part of the elderly person. This is usually the real tip-off that things are amiss.

Marie, for instance, a fabulous cook, could suddenly no longer follow her own handwritten recipes. Nelson, an aging golf pro, would go out to buy the newspaper and get lost on his way home. Rita worked with numbers all her life at an actuarial firm. One day she discovered almost overnight that she was unable to do the simple arithmetic necessary for computing a compound interest problem. Jose, a high-paid financial executive, started wearing different color socks to the office and consistently forgetting to tuck in his stylish shirts.

Cooking, walking home, adding and subtracting, and dressing are deeply familiar activities that most of us do impeccably every day without a second thought. People who find such tasks suddenly unmanageable or confusing are usually people in trouble.

Thus the first possible danger signs of AD or a demential disease include these:

- An inability to perform familiar tasks
- Trouble organizing and sequencing familiar information: knowing where something goes, how it goes, and why it goes there
- Changes in habitual behavior patterns
- Gradual memory loss

Include several other possible symptoms as well: the loss of a viable time sense, indulgence in embarrassing social behavior (speaking too loudly at a restaurant, climbing up on the counter at a department store, etc.), and a sudden inability to retain information that is usually easily learned. These generalize to two more danger signs:

- Sudden, dramatic lack of social inhibition
- Diminution of reason and problem-solving abilities and an inability to adapt to simple change

It is sometimes said that in the early stages of AD, patients are unaware that they are having problems. Margaret was one such case. But this is not inevitably true. Some people are very aware, so much so that it is they, not the spouse or children, who insist on a visit to the physician. Note too that contrary to popular belief, no absolute correlation can be made between present symptoms and past tendencies. Even though Allen has always been a generous man and even a spendthrift, this does not mean he will squander his money even more freely when in the grips of Alzheimer's. To the contrary, when Allen developed Alzheimer's disease he became aggressively closefisted and even paranoid about his finances. On the other hand, it is also common among demented persons to see normal behavior patterns turn exaggerated and even psychotic. Nana S., for instance, was always a neat and spotless person during her fifty or more years of married life. When she developed dementia, her wholesome love of tidiness became a mad compulsion, and she spent most of her day wiping the furniture and scrubbing the floors.

What about emotions? What changes might you expect to see in this critical area? Inappropriate suspiciousness, for one ("I didn't give you permission to wear my sweatshirt!" "Someone stole my cuff links again!"). Sudden anger and unaccountable upsets over ordinary events (one woman cried every time she brushed her teeth). Lowered frustration levels (a carpenter with dementia flew into a tantrum when he missed a nail or mismeasured a saw cut; a cashier screamed at her customers even though it was she who was consistently miscounting change). And finally, any type of bizarre, abnormal, and inappropriate emotional behavior (laughing without provocation; delivering declarations of love to the grocer; breaking into song in the middle of a business meeting). So our final additions to the list of possible warning symptoms include these:

- Increased suspiciousness and paranoia
- Inability to control anger, rage, and frustration
- Frequent catastrophic outbursts
- Sudden and dramatic changes in the emotional persona

This inventory is enough to help you make preliminary judgments concerning whether or not to seek professional help.

If you do decide to see a physician, however, realize that you are still a long way from a diagnosis of Alzheimer's and that before such a diagnosis can be suggested, a number of alternatives must be ruled out. Such determinations can, of course, only be made by the doctor. But you can help.

2

Diagnosing Alzheimer's and Getting the Most Out of Medical Care

Before the First Doctor's Visit

For your own peace of mind, and so that you will be able to deal with your loved one's symptomatology with greater authority, it is generally suggested that you become familiar with the medical principles on which an Alzheimer's diagnosis is made, and that you do so before your first visit to a clinic or physician.

To begin, let us reiterate that AD can never be diagnosed with total confidence and that no infallible lab tests have yet been developed to verify its presence in the brain. Given these limits, a differential diagnosis must be approached not by testing for AD itself but by ruling out all other ailments that produce AD-like symptoms, a method based on a battery of neurological, medical, and psychological test procedures.

The diagnostic procedure for AD is thus really an elaborate process of elimination, a so-called diagnosis of exclusion, and sometimes a lengthy one at that. This process of elimination involves two basic steps: first, determining if the patient is suffering from a real dementia such as Alzheimer's disease or from a dementia look-alike, and second, once it is established that a dementia is present, determining the kind of dementia the person is suffering from.

Let us start with the dementia look-alikes. Generally, and in somewhat oversimplified terms perhaps, two categories of dementia look-alikes are most likely to turn up: delirium and depression.

Delirium

Delirium is a state of mental confusion and diminished consciousness characterized by an acute, rapid onset of symptoms. It can be recognized by such behavioral patterns as these:

- Confusion, forgetfulness, and disassociation
- Marked reduction of attention span
- Sleep disturbances
- Fluctuations between restlessness and apathy
- Delusions and hallucinations

Ordinarily triggered by dramatic conditions such as fevers, toxic poisoning, metabolic disturbances, and medications, delirium can likewise be brought on by malnutrition or sudden shocks to the organism. In especially fragile persons, a change in location will sometimes produce symptoms. In others it will be the result of withdrawal from addictive substances or adverse reactions to drugs.

Although delirium causes symptoms similar to those found in AD, the two conditions are relatively easy for an alert physician to tell apart.

The primary characteristic differentiating delirium from dementia is that delirium almost always comes on abruptly and aggressively, sometimes in a matter of hours, and often with little prior warning. Dementia, by contrast, especially Alzheimer's dementia, has a relatively slow and insidious onset. Also, delirious persons suffer from a kind of clouded, dazed state of consciousness that waxes and wanes throughout the day; dementia sufferers maintain relatively constant levels of awareness throughout the day and do not ordinarily appear to be suffering from lowered consciousness per se.

Depression

Depression can often be hard to differentiate from dementia, and mistaking the first condition for the second is probably the most common medical misdiagnosis (it is estimated that before 1982, one-third of patients diagnosed as having Alzheimer's disease were actually suffering from depression; it is also believed that approximately twenty percent of *all* persons over sixty-five in the United States suffer from some degree of depression).

Depressed people may mix up their words, the same as demented persons. They will display the same glazed, abstracted expression. Or, conversely, they may become restless and disoriented and even pace in the manner of a demented patient. Memory slips: Sufferers will suddenly blank out on their home address or forget how to knot a necktie. They may stop eating; they may become cranky and disinclined to talk. They may become easily fatigued and lose interest in everyday fun and events—all changes that sound ominously like dementia pathology.

Still, there are tangible differences between depression and AD, and these will often be as apparent to the family as they are to the physician. Clinically speaking, depressed persons show a markedly positive response to medications, particularly to antidepressants and mood enhancers. Observable positive changes in depression can be fostered by psychotherapy or even by improved life circumstances at home and in the office. The depressed person will blank out on a name or address, perhaps, but may remember it later. He or she may forget a portion of an address (or of a name, an incident, a telephone conversation) but not the whole thing. Not so the demented person. He or she may never again recall the missing piece of information. It is gone now forever. Unlike depression, the symptoms of AD are progressive, nonresponsive to psychiatric intervention, and absolutely irreversible.

Depressed persons, as a rule, are extremely aware of their slipping capacities. AD sufferers may be less tuned in to adverse mental changes and may not worry about them, even when they know something is amiss. Or they may often deny symptoms entirely, even while depressed persons make a peevish point of reporting each and every one of their recent mental goofs. A depressed person's knack for recalling the minutiae of daily life is waning, yes. But such persons forget far less frequently than they *think* they do, and when asked to enumerate the kinds of items that do slip their minds—inherently forgettable things, usually, like keys, appointments, names, book titles—they will recall an inventory down to the nth detail. With AD sufferers it's different; they tend, as it were, to forget what they forget.

"People who come to me complaining of memory loss," explains David Kamlet, M.D., a specialist in geriatric medicine and staff member of Bellevue Hospital's Geriatric Ambulatory Care Program, "usually are having depression, not dementia." He continues:

> People with Alzheimer's don't often come in at first complaining of memory loss. Something else brings them in, like confusion or weird mental symptoms. In addition, if there's been an abrupt onset of these symptoms over the past few weeks or so, this probably also means depression. If it's short-term memory, not long-term memory, that's another indication of depression.

After delirium, depression, and several less probable dementia look-alikes are ruled out, the physician is faced with the even more formidable task of assessing exactly what type of dementia is actually to blame for the symptoms. Most important, this determination will tell whether the dementia is reversible or irreversible, and hence treatable or untreatable.

As mentioned in Chapter 1, more than sixty reversible forms of dementia afflict the human mind, and physicians must be aware of at least the most prominent of these when making a differential diagnosis. Dementia can be caused, for example, by a reaction to medication: A single dose of a drug such as Valium stays in the system for as long as a week and in certain cases can turn the user into an Alzheimer's-like zombie. Persons on sedative drugs, hypnotics, sleep medications, anticonvulsants, and antipsychotics can all present dementialike symptoms.

Dehydration, low sodium or low magnesium, thyroid problems, pernicious anemia, Addison's disease, and liver or kidney failure must all be considered during the course of the examination. Other possible causes include nutritional disorders—pellagra and thiamine deficiency can both produce dementia, and people have actually been institutionalized for a supposed psychosis when in fact they were suffering from an inability to process vitamin B_{12}. Other possible reasons for dementia include hyperthyroidism or hypothyroidism, head injuries, AIDS and general viral infections (even small urinary tract infections can occasionally produce cognitive disorders), lupus erythematosus, toxic or alcoholic poisoning, psychiatric disorders (such as schizophrenia), brain tumors, hormonal abnormalities, electrolyte imbalance, and neurosyphilis.

After all the entries on the long list of dementia look-alikes have been checked off in this diagnosis of exclusion and after it is clear that the ailment is not due to a transient or nonprogressive pathology, it must be assumed that the problem at hand is indeed chronic dementia, progressive, irreversible, and incurable, and that, except for certain drugs that palliate symptoms, the disorder is medically untreatable.

What ailments fall into the category of irreversible chronic dementias? First, neurological disorders such as Pick's and Creutzfeldt-Jakob disease must be mentioned, but these sicknesses are seldom seen. Huntington's disease and Parkinson's disease produce symptoms that are fairly easy to tell apart from Alzheimer's.

This leaves one last possible disease to be seriously considered before a diagnosis of AD can be suggested, a debilitating and nonreversible senile disorder known as *multi-infarct dementia,* or MID.

An infarct is a small, localized cluster of brain cells that has been damaged or destroyed by a sudden deprivation of blood. In the specific case of multi-infarct dementia, cell death results from a number of small, undetectable strokes that occur over a prolonged period of time and leave a graveyard of dead neural material in their wake.

As with AD patients, MID dramatically reduces a person's mental and social capabilities. Speech becomes affected, as does judgment, emotion, motor coordination, and common sense.

Despite the similarities between them, however, AD and MID are discernible to a practiced professional eye. First, MID tends to affect persons between forty and sixty years of age, whereas AD does not usually manifest until around the sixty-fifth year. In the lab, CAT scans can sometimes pick up physiological differences between these two disorders, and so will radioisotope studies of cerebral blood flow. MID, moreover, has a more abrupt onset than Alzheimer's disease and develops in discrete steps—quantum leaps, if you will—or, conversely, it may remain at a particular level of development for years, even decades. AD, by contrast, marches ahead slowly, inevitably, inexorably, without remaining very long at one particular point, without responding to preventive measures, and without either slowing or accelerating its pace.

Tests and Examinations: What to Expect During the Clinical Diagnosis

During the 1970s the accuracy of differential diagnosis for dementia was woefully inadequate. Many poignant cases occurred in which persons were informed that they did not have Alzheimer's disease when in fact they did—and vice versa. Finally, several years ago a group of neurologists met and formulated a new approach to dementia diagnosis that they believed would be far more effective. Their conclusions revolutionized doctors' diagnostic approach to dementia. Thanks to the new method, the accuracy of AD diagnosis now ranges between eighty and ninety percent.

CRITERIA FOR CLINICAL DIAGNOSIS OF ALZHEIMER'S DISEASE

Criteria of Probable *Alzheimer's Disease*
> Dementia on clinical examination, documented by mental status tests and confirmed by neuropsychologic tests
> Deficits in two or more cognitive areas

Progressive worsening of memory and other cognitive functions

No disturbance of consciousness

Onset between the ages of forty and ninety, usually after age sixty-five

Absence of systemic or brain disorders that in themselves could account for the progressive memory and cognitive deficits

Evidence to Support Diagnosis of Probable *Alzheimer's Disease*

Progressive deterioration of specific cognitive functions (e.g., language, motor skills, perception)

Impairment of activities of daily living and altered behavior patterns

Family history of similar disorders (especially if confirmed pathologically)

Normal lumbar puncture results

Normal or nonspecific (e.g., slow-wave) changes in EEG

Progressive cerebral atrophy on serial CAT scans

Features Consistent with Probable *Alzheimer's Disease After Exclusion of Other Causes of Dementia*

Plateaus in the progression of the illness

Associated symptoms: depression, insomnia, incontinence, delusions, illusions, hallucinations, catastrophic reactions (verbal, emotional, physical), sexual disorders, weight loss

Other neurologic abnormalities (especially in advanced cases) including increased muscle tone, myoclonus, and gait disorders

Seizures (in advanced cases)

Features Inconsistent with Probable *Alzheimer's Disease that Make Diagnosis Uncertain or Unlikely*

Sudden apoplectic onset

Focal neurologic findings, such as hemiparesis, sensory loss, visual field defects, and early incoordination

Early seizures or gait disturbances

Criteria for Clinical Diagnosis of Possible *Alzheimer's Disease*

Dementia syndrome with variations in the onset, presentation, or course, in the absence of other disorders that in themselves may cause dementia

Dementia associated with a second system or brain disorder that would be sufficient to produce dementia but is not considered the prime cause

Single, gradually progressive, and severe cognitive deficit in the absence of an identifiable cause

Criteria for Diagnosis of Definite *Alzheimer's Disease*

Criteria for probable Alzheimer's disease plus evidence from biopsy or autopsy

Employing a three-part strategy that called for medical testing and a physical exam, a thorough medical history, and a battery of psychological tests, this method was published in several neurological journals in 1984 and has since set the standard for AD diagnostic methodology in the United States.

Based on the principles developed in the "Criteria for Clinical Diagnosis," all persons suspected of having a dementia will thus be given a three-part examination consisting of a physical exam, a review of past medical history, and a series of psychological tests. First, the physical exam.

The Physical Examination

All persons suspected of cognitive impairment will first be given a checkup by a doctor to assess their state of physical and neurological health. The checkup will consist of the usual clinical measures: listening to the heart and lungs, reflex testing, and so on, and the findings will be supplemented by a series of standard lab tests. These tests will in all likelihood include the following:

• Electroencephalogram (EEG). A series of electrodes are attached to the person's scalp, and the brain's electrical impulses are recorded. If these impulses register irregular patterns, this may indicate a brain injury of some kind, such as a stroke, a head trauma, or a tumor. Though electroencephalograms are painless, having electrodes attached to one's skull is a disconcerting experience, especially if a person is already showing signs of dementialike behavior. When the equipment is being attached, stay near the elderly person and talk reassuringly to him or her until the test starts. Sometimes it will take several minutes before the person is willing to begin. Just be patient and keep the reassurances coming that the test is painless. It is.

• Computerized axial tomography (CAT scan). The patient lies on a table, his or her head is enclosed in a space-age, helmetlike affair, and multiple X rays are taken of different areas in the brain. These images are then read and evaluated by a computer. Though a CAT scan cannot diagnose AD, it is capable of recognizing other dementia-causing problems such as brain tumors, strokes, clots, or hydrocephalus, and thus, like the electroencephalogram, it can help eliminate Alzheimer's disease from the list of possible ailments.

At one time brain scans required an injection of radioactive dye, but this unpleasant procedure is no longer necessary; and the X ray is now completely painless. A claustrophobic person, however, already disoriented by the hospital environment, will still be ill at ease with the CAT scan apparatus, and sometimes no amount of coaxing will convince the patient to climb onto this "contraption." Though CAT scans (and a related technology called magnetic resonance imaging, which employs magnetic beams instead of X rays) are routinely used today for the diagnosis of brain problems, it is not one hundred percent necessary for patients to have one, especially if they are excessively intimidated by all this looming machinery.

• Laboratory tests. Several lab tests will be ordered including blood chemistry checks for liver and kidney ailments plus a complete blood count (CBC) and a sedimentation rate (ESR) to locate possible infections and even hidden cancer. Most of the time these tests require nothing more than finger pricks to draw blood and are usually not upsetting to patients.

Urine samples will then be taken to check for diabetes and viral infections, and vitamin B_{12} levels will be checked, along with thyroid function. If there is any indication that the dementia is produced by neurosyphilis, a venereal disease test will also be ordered. Occasionally, a spinal tap is taken to evaluate the chemistry of the cerebrospinal fluid, but its value is somewhat dubious in this situation, and many doctors do not recommend it. An electrocardiograph and routine X rays may be administered to determine the person's general level of health. Chest X rays will rule out possible TB as a source of dementia.

• Folic acid test. Finally, doctors may look for deficiencies of folic acid as a sign of hidden alcoholism. Most professionals now believe that chronic drinking can produce a recurring dementia.

The Medical History

Doctors will next wish to conduct a medical history interview with the elderly person, and here caregivers can really help. Why? Because as a rule, there will be so many distractions in the doctor's office that the elderly person may not be particularly sharp during these sessions. Facts will be forgotten, significant questions will go unasked, important concerns unmentioned. This means that you as caregiver should be prepared to raise or answer the questions that the elderly person cannot handle him or herself. You will be, as it were, the stand-in memory.

The following list of questions, typical of what the doctor may ask you and the patient during the medical history interview, should be studied and contemplated before the first visit. Of course, each doctor will have particular points of inquiry, but you will find this list to be quite representative.

- Describe the first signs of abnormality that you (or the patient) noticed in the patient's behavior. Carefully depict all present symptoms.
- Is there any past history of heart disease or stroke?
- For how long a period of time have the symptoms been apparent? When did they begin? Were they triggered by a particular experience or illness?
- Has the patient recently or in the past sustained a serious head injury? Have the symptoms become worse or have they remained constant?
- In what order did the symptoms appear? All at once? One at a time? Did they come on abruptly or gradually? Did they take days, weeks, or months to become evident enough for you to seek help? Does the elderly person have any of the following symptoms? If so, describe them in detail.

1. Memory loss: Does the person deny having memory loss? Does he or she blame the forgetfulness on other persons or on improbable causes? ("The alarm clock rang so loud," one older person remarked in all seriousness, "it made me forget it was time to get up.")

2. Catastrophic emotional outbursts: Are these reactions triggered by situations that did not previously bother the person? Do they center on trivial or incidental events?

3. Mood swings: Does the person seem depressed? Is he or she listless and apathetic? Restless? Agitated much of the time?

4. Personality changes: Has any sudden, dramatic, or atypical change occurred?

5. Uninhibited behavior: Has the person demonstrated uncharacteristically abnormal sexual behavior or antisocial conduct?

6. Delusions: Has the person become unreasonably or uncharacteristically suspicious?

7. Language problems: Is the person forgetting words?

8. Difficulty with previously easy tasks: Does the person have difficulty taking a telephone message, getting dressed, balancing a checkbook, keeping score in a card game, or taking a shower?

9. Concentration ability: Has this declined? Has the person ever become lost or spacially disoriented?

- Has anyone else in your family demonstrated symptoms similar to those that are bothering the patient? Is there any history of neurological disease in your family? If so, what?
- Does the patient have a past history of psychiatric disease of any kind: mania, depression, schizophrenia? Is there a family history of mental disease?
- Has the person's condition been studied by a doctor already? If so, what was the diagnosis? Has the patient undergone tests for this problem? Is he or she presently taking medication for this problem?
- What general medications is the person taking? Be sure to state the brand name or generic name, the strength, the frequency of dose, and whether the drug is in capsule or pill form, over-the-counter or prescription. It is also a good idea to bring the medication with you for the doctor to see.
- What is the elderly person's present state of health? Does he or she exercise? Smoke? Drink a lot of coffee or tea? What are his or her eating habits? Has the person suffered from any chronic ailments over the past years? If so, describe. Has he or she had any recent surgery?
- Does the person drink alcohol heavily? If so, describe the patterns.
- What is the elderly person's profession? Does it involve toxic chemicals or wastes of any kind? Does the person have hobbies (such as model making) that require the use of strong glues and fixatives?

Mental Status Testing

Finally, the elderly person's cognitive capacities will be assessed via a series of psychological and neurological tests. These tests will sometimes determine a great deal about the person. They can, for instance, help doctors make the difficult differentiation between dementia, delirium, and depression. In certain instances they will also help examiners zero in on which particular kind of dementia is at work and how advanced the ailment has become.

Expect patients to be given one or more mental status questionnaires. Usually these questionnaires are terse and to the point. But though they may appear simplistic, even a mentally normal person will occasionally flub an answer or two.

Finally, persons will be examined neurologically and will be given a number of simple tasks to perform such as describing, with eyes closed, which of their hands the examiner is touching to which of their cheeks (right hand to left cheek, right hand to right cheek, etc.). More than five errors is grounds for suspicion of dementia. Language abilities, coordination, memory, logic, abstract reasoning, attention span, and several other cognitive skills may all be tested, both physically and via written exams. The results of all these tests are then evaluated, leading, ideally, to a clear-cut diagnosis.

Waiting

At the end of these rounds of physical and psychological probing, a fairly clear portrait of the person's condition and cognitive health will usually—but not always—emerge.

Don't be surprised, for instance, if the physician calls you back for further testing. Or if after waiting several weeks you are informed that the results are still inconclusive and that the doctor cannot be sure of anything until more tests are made. Dementia is a treacherous and illusive ailment. Researchers are just beginning to figure out how to measure and assess it and to understand how it develops in the human cortex. An honest physician will pull no punches with you on this score and will certainly not pretend to possess anything approaching surety as to the diagnosis.

Sometimes, for instance, the doctor will need more data to work with and will send you to another specialist for further lab work. Sometimes he or she will want you to bring the person back in, say, six months to a year when, presumably, the symptoms will be more developed and easier to read. Sometimes he or she may simply be stumped, telling you the somewhat disconcerting news that there is simply no way at this time to be certain of anything. Consider this a mercy, by the way. Better uncertainty than a positive diagnosis of chronic dementia.

Reactions to the Diagnosis: Yours and the Patient's

If something is broken, we get it fixed. If one solution fizzles, we come up with another. That's just the way it is in the modern, can-do world.

But with Alzheimer's disease, there are simply no alternatives, no fixes, no cures:

"Your spouse has Alzheimer's disease, Mrs. Johnson."

"What kind of treatment will it require, doctor?"

"I'm afraid at the present time there is no treatment, Mrs. Johnson."

"Surely there must be *something* you can do."

"Other than sedating him when he gets agitated, I'm afraid there's not a great deal."

"But there must be—*something!*"

The phrase "Surely there must be *something!*" echoes in thousands of medical examining rooms each year, always, no doubt, in the same amazed and totally frustrated tone of voice. Hear several caregivers describe their emotions when first hearing that a loved one had AD:

Sue: After all that waiting. All that waiting. We had spent long nights up with Mom. She couldn't sleep. Or eat. She was acting really weird and it just wasn't like her to get up from the dinner table and walk away. She'd been doing things like fidgeting with her fork and dropping it and not picking it up. My brothers and sisters are all married, I'm the only child at home, with Pop. We got so worried but Pop didn't want to take her to the doctors. After all the postponing, with Mom getting worse-acting anyway, we took her, and finally got the word after a lot of tests: Alzheimer's disease. I'd never heard of it. The doctor explained to me what it was and I thought I was going to vomit right there, it sounded so terrible. I didn't know what to do. I looked at Pop and he had big tears in his eyes, and was looking at Mom who was fidgeting in the corner with her fingers. She seemed not to care anything about it at all. Just out of it. I myself wanted to crawl under the couch in the examining room and hide.

Lester: I heard the word "Alzheimer" mentioned about my wife of forty-two happy years, and I guess when it came out of that doctor's mouth I wanted to punch him in that mouth that had described these words. It was his fault. All those tests and the money we'd spent, and what did we have to show for it? A diagnosis of a deadly disease. Damn! *He* had caused it, I said to myself. It was his fault, he gave her the disease. I knew it was irrational and crazy. But at that moment my world caved in and I'm a big man, strong. I had to do everything I could to stop myself from grabbing the doctor by the throat and making him take back what he'd just said about this Alzheimer's disease thing.

Louise: Leslie [my brother] took the news that he had Alzheimer's disease with the kind of great dignity with which he takes all news, good and bad. He thanked the doctor and I took him home to his apartment. I stayed at his apartment with him that evening and we talked, and he seemed composed and resigned, but then in the middle of dinner he dropped a bit of his dinner on the floor and just broke up crying. I had a hard time settling him down after that. I promised I'd come visit every day for the next week or so. That seemed to be a comfort. We talked about getting a live-in nurse. He doubted whether his insurance would pay for it but I said it would. I have some savings too. That helped him get his bearings. I know he secretly wanted me to come live there with him but he was too proud to say it. The next few months after he got the news he was a worried and distracted man suffering from a terrible disease. And only in his early sixties. I wished the doctor had told me and not him. Or at least broken the news to him more slowly. He had become very agitated and ill at ease since that day.

Processing the Information

Once a positive diagnosis has been made, the first question you must come to grips with is whether or not the person knows the truth. The second is, if not, should he or she be told?

There is no magic pointer to guide you through this difficult choice, but many health care professionals agree that it is usually in the best interests of all parties to inform persons of their diagnosis at the start. For some, simply learning that they have an identifiable disease and that they are not "losing their minds" is a comfort. As long as the person is at least somewhat mentally competent, moreover, playing the tricky game of dissimulation will produce a tangled web indeed. Oh, we can tell a spouse or a parent that her forgetfulness is due to advancing age and nothing more. But as the days pass, as her memory and her behavior become more and more obviously aberrant, it gets tougher and tougher for family members caught up in the terrible conspiracy of denial to continue their cheerful assurances that everything is fine, just fine. Only confusion and anxiety can result from such intimate pretending.

It is better to lay all cards on the table. If persons are in the early stages of the disease, you can talk to them about it directly. They will understand the facts and, ideally, will be willing to share their feelings about it with you. Make it clear to the person that he or she is suffering from a brain disease that affects memory, coordination, and speech but involves no pain or suffering. Many people will want to know if they are "going crazy." Explain that they have a disease, not a psychosis, and that there are medicines that can reduce the level of anxiety should they become especially agitated or upset. Persons will also ask about the future and about whether or not they will be "stuck" in an institution.

Assure them that as things stand now, they will not be abandoned or put away.

Be honest, simple, and direct. Make it clear to your elderly loved ones that they still have time to lead relatively normal lives, that no one is exactly sure how long AD takes to develop, and that you, the caregiver (and other family members, if such be the case), will be on hand to help. Describe a few of the dementia-related problems that may occur during the course of daily life, such as undue forgetfulness or an inability to balance a checkbook. Give specific examples whenever possible, and explain how you as caregiver will help. Do not, however, volunteer more information than the person wishes to hear. For some, a little disclosure is a lot. Others will not want to hear anything at all on the subject, at least for now. So be it—you have done your duty, and the rest is up to the patient.

The diagnosis of dementia is a truly agonizing experience for everyone. But it will have to be faced, if not today then tomorrow, or the day after, or the day after that. When all is said and done, telling sick persons the truth right away tends to cut through a number of potential entanglements and to dispel the need for prevarication and subterfuge later on. It also allows loved ones time to tie up the loose ends of life and to figure out how they can best use their remaining time. In the long run, open disclosure is usually the best way.

Dealing with Denial

The first few days after they got the news I guess I just sort of didn't want to deal with it. A cold silence reigned around their household. A terrible black cloud was over everything, but nobody wanted to talk about it. Dad kept in his room most of the time, and Mom kept to hers. I could hear crying come out through the door sometimes when I passed both their rooms. One day when we were over to my parents' house for dinner and I decided to just cut through this conspiracy of silence and bring it up. I expected that Dad and Mom would clam up. We were all sitting around the table, I remember it so well, and I asked Dad what he was doing about his Alzheimer's disease now. For a second he looked at me as if I'd just struck him. Then he started talking, slowly at first, then it all gushed out—the sedatives, the side effects, the worry that he'd take the wrong medicines, his worry about leaving Mom to hold the bag financially, his fears of setting the house on fire when he lit his cigars. It just kept pouring out. We talked for several hours that night.

This is the son of an Alzheimer's sufferer speaking, and his experience is typical. Immediately after the diagnosis, dementia victims are often reluctant to discuss their disease. Some deny it entirely; others insist it is just a passing phase. Yet this attitude can change in a few months' time, and the afflicted person may often become frankly and openly communicative. When someone is suffering from a terminal ailment like AD, there is not a whole lot caretakers can do to make things any better for the suffering person; however, there are things they can do to prevent things from getting worse. Letting the person talk, question, and vent feelings are three of the most important.

As a general rule, people who receive terrible news tend to process it in stages. First comes the shock: "What?" Then the denial: "No, not me!" Then the anger: "Why me?" Then the dejection and desolation: "Poor me!" And finally, the acceptance: "Yes, me." Though these stages do not follow one another neatly and while they sometimes come all at once or in abrupt staccato, they *do* come for just about everyone. Consequently, it is one of the caregiver's many jobs to help the stricken person sort out these feelings, to work the person through this harsh twist of fate until the affliction can be accepted as part of reality. One demented individual, a textbook salesman named George, tended to wake up mornings in a state of denial, telling his wife that he had finally "licked this thing" and that he no longer needed his medication. By noon the same man was deeply depressed and had to be coaxed to eat lunch. "I can't stand it," he would cry. "I can't stand knowing I'm going to become a dumb vegetable soon!" Finally, toward evening, like clockwork, he would begin to reminisce about his past, announcing that he'd had a wonderful life and proclaiming that even though he had AD, there was still lots of life left in him. The same pattern repeated itself every day.

Sometimes demented persons will not be mentally focused enough to comprehend the full significance of the diagnosis. Yet they know that something is out of joint, and they grope for reassurance. Give it to them.

In other cases persons know the truth but may not want to bring the matter up. They wish to spare *you.* If this is the case, assure them that you are indeed aware of how things are and that you are more than happy to discuss matters at any time. "The best thing I could ever do for Tony," an elderly woman told us about her recently deceased husband of forty-one years, "was to go with him on his walks after lunch and to remind him once again who I was, why we were here on his favorite forest trail, and that, yes, he was sick but that I loved him and would be with him all the time. That always seemed to make him quiet down and become happy."

If persons actively wish to deny their ailment or to pretend that it is only temporary, it is not necessarily your job to set them straight. Sometimes denial is the only possible accommodation in the face of agony. Indeed, denial may not always be such a terrible thing; at times it can be a downright comfort for those who invoke it. It depends on the circumstances. You will have to judge for yourself. However, you as caregiver would be well advised to avoid the pitfalls of denial *yourself*, whatever the situation, and to face matters squarely from the beginning. Remember, pretending that this disease is not as serious as the doctors tell you; that nature will heal it in time; that with hard work you and the person can lick it; that no one can predict the future, so why try; that a cure is just around the corner; that the disease has been misdiagnosed; that this nightmare will go away on its own and that one morning you will wake up and the skies will be blue again—these and a thousand other wish fulfillment fantasies are only traps that prevent you from adequately preparing for the long haul ahead and dull your ability to look after the sick person's needs and your own. Burying your head in the sand, in this instance, will only make you blind.

When you do speak about the diagnosis with patients who are still rational, invoke the "glass is half full" approach: Stress the fact that there is still time, still many things to be done, still places to visit, tasks to be accomplished, life to be lived. It will be a comfort for persons to know that a specific caregiver has been designated to help look after their legal and financial particulars and to take care of them when they become incapacitated. One of the ways we can serve sick persons best is to work out with them in advance the details of their insurance, their future medical care, their private affairs, their finances—Chapter 9 will cover these matters in full.

Digesting the News

A diagnosis of dementia will elicit an amazingly wide range of shock reactions from patients and caregivers alike. For some, the news is a prognosis worse than death, a verdict of zombielike existence in which family members perceive their loved one as already a kind of quasi-functional puppet whose inner person has faded away and who is un-reachable on any level. Others take a cool, wait-and-see attitude, hoping that there will be an angle to play, some alternative medication, some magical ace in the hole that makes it all OK. For others, learning about dementia sharpens the resolve to fight, to live each remaining hour, to stay alive. For still others, the denial process is set into motion: Families gloss over the hard facts of the case. They play down the disease's importance and attempt to continue living as if nothing is different.

But something *is* different, and it will be different from now on, the person's condition creeping, year to year, relentlessly downward along the graph of mental deterioration. This is stark stuff for any of us to accept, and for some it is too big a hunk of reality to swallow at a single bite. Space is needed to think things over. Time is required to digest it all.

Allow yourself and your loved one this time and space. Allow yourself the luxury of adjustment, of thinking things over and carefully assessing the next move. Now is *not* the time to do anything rash or extravagant. Perhaps your first impulse will be to get a second opinion. Is this wise? Unless you have good cause to think otherwise, why be in too much of a hurry to rush out for another diagnosis—and then another and another and another? Most M.D.'s, especially specialists who deal with dementia every day, tend to be fairly accurate in their assessments, and diagnostic methods are improving all the time. Down the line, after some time has passed and you have been able to assess the sick person's condition yourself and judge whether the doctor's prognosis is bearing itself out or not, if you still feel strongly that the sickness has been misdiagnosed, it may be time for another professional to take a look. Just beware of what Marion M. called the "second opinion circus":

> *Marion:* When we heard that Herbert, my husband, had Alzheimer's disease, we didn't want to believe it. We bought some books about Alzheimer's and noticed that Herbert did not have all the classic symptoms that were mentioned there. An army buddy of Herbert's warned us that Alzheimer's disease is often misdiagnosed. We figured that the doctor must have made a mistake. So we went to a psychiatrist out of state who came highly recommended. We thought Herbert was just depressed or something. Luckily, this doctor was an upright man and after several sessions with Herb he said he honestly thought the problem was physical, not psychological. We'd better have it looked at by a doctor. We went back into the second opinion circus again, to another doctor, and after a long time and a lot of money he told us the same thing, that all signs pointed to my husband's having Alzheimer's disease. I believed it by now but Herbert didn't—wouldn't, didn't really want to—and to make a long story short, we ended up going to three more specialists. Of course, it takes some time to examine a person for these diseases and after a while his symptoms were becoming pretty plain. I was in charge and I guided him away from getting more medical opinions. It seemed pretty clear that what the doctors said was right.

Above all, bear in mind that panic and despair are blind alleys for *everyone* and that if you throw in the towel in the beginning, when the condition is still manageable, the person will quickly lose hope too. Instead, take stock of the situation and try your hardest, your absolute hardest, to remember that there is still time remaining for you and your loved one to live meaningful days together and that there *are* things you can do to soften the blow of the diagnosis, things that on the one hand will help you to detour despair and on the other avoid unrealistic flights of denial fantasy. Here are some experience-proven suggestions.

1. Be Prepared for an Aftershock

During the first postexamination meeting with the physician, when the diagnosis is being delivered, caregivers and patients alike report that they often remain outwardly calm and composed. Then, hours or even days later, the full significance of the news hits like a Mack truck. Some people begin to shake or have palpitations. They feel faint, suffer anxiety and disorientation attacks, or describe symptoms of deep depression. When Roger L. was told that he had MID and that the ailment was progressive and incurable, he cried uncontrollably for several weeks. When Luis de P. was told that his wife had Alzheimer's, he walked the streets aimlessly for two nights in a row.

If aftershock symptoms plague you in the first days or weeks after the diagnosis, know that they are transitory and normal. You are not going crazy. You are OK. Talking about these feelings with friends or other family members, a therapist, or your doctor will help. So will the simple passing of time.

2. Learn About the Disease

Knowledge helps, and health care professionals can be crucial partners in your education. Try not to sit passively in the consultation room when your loved one's condition is discussed. Ask questions. Find out everything you can about the disease. Read books. Consult the medical literature. Talk to other people who have nursed a demented person or who know something about the subject. Seek out social workers, nurses, home care aids, and other professionals who have dealt with dementia in the past. Keep a pad handy to jot down queries as they occur; they will. Before you visit any health care professionals, make sure you have all major questions clearly lined up in your mind. Writing them down beforehand always helps.

3. *Doctors Are Principal Resources—Choose Them Wisely*

Don't be shy about eliciting your physician's help. Keep his or her phone number handy at all times. Make contact whenever you need advice or support. Health care professionals worth their salt will take the time, especially at the beginning, to go over the whys and wherefores of dementia, to discuss all medical options firsthand, and to provide emotional support when it's asked for.

Dr. David Kamlet, whom we met in Chapter 1, describes the services that he, as a specialist treating Alzheimer's disease and related dementias, believes a good doctor should provide for the family of patients:

> First of all, the kind of doctor you want treating Alzheimer's is a doctor with academic affiliations, either board certified or on the staff of hospitals where they are obliged to be involved in teaching. Someone in contact with recent medical literature. Someone who knows all the latest-breaking developments in the field. Avoid doctors who are very optimistic and promise the world; and avoid doctors who are the other way around, who throw up their hands and tell you there's no hope, that it's all a *fait accompli.*
>
> After the preliminary diagnosis is made and after everything that can be done is done, a good doctor should now concentrate on the caregivers. The doctor should see that their needs are met, both emotional and physical. The biggest thing here is encouragement. Letting the caregiver know that she is doing a good job. Also, caregivers need to vent. They need to get out their misplaced feelings and their guilts. Alzheimer's patients, you see, lose their inhibitions and say the most terrible things to caregivers. Insults, nasty accusations, terrible stabs and slurs. This can make family members who are giving their all to the patient very depressed, and it may contribute to the development of secret hate feelings for the patient. The caregiver must consequently be reminded that the patient is *sick* and that it is the disease that is speaking so antagonistically, not the person.
>
> Finally, a doctor should serve as an intermediary with the family. Many times a doctor can do things that others can't simply because of his particular position. Using my influence, I try to take the burden off one particular family member and divide it among several. Sometimes an outsider such as the physician is needed to take an authoritative position like this, to say, "Look, from my perspective this is not good. This person needs a break. Her health is being threatened. It's your responsibility to share this burden if you

don't want her to end up in a nursing home herself." I say "she," by the way, because they've discovered that ninety percent of caregivers in this country are female.

4. Find Out What to Expect

One way of gaining a small but precious foothold of control over the future is to acquire as much medical knowledge as possible concerning the kinds of behavior, both physical and emotional, you can expect from the ailing person at different points in the disease and then to plan accordingly.

First, there is the question of determining how demented the person is at this particular time. Although it is impossible to quantify this matter precisely, several fairly accurate behavioral rating scales have been worked out to determine dementia disability degrees.

Having an approximate notion of a person's present level of dementia, it is informative as well to know how the person's condition will tend to develop as time passes. We say "tend" because each case is different. Several years ago it was fashionable to claim that Alzheimer's disease developed in a series of four or five clear-cut stages, but further research has shown that AD's progress cannot be mapped so predictably. At the same time, however, a very general schedule of development does seem to occur among a majority of patients, and knowledge of this very approximate timetable will help you and your loved one maximize the quality time that remains. General stages of dementia run generally as follows:

A. *The early stages:* The early stages of the disease, as we have seen, are often typified by physical and characterological changes that parody and exaggerate the normal process of aging. Patients forget easily. They become lost or disoriented easily and seem to lose their capacity for learning anything new. Apathy and listlessness set in. Ordinary, everyday words are forgotten. Fatigue comes more quickly than before. Intellectual judgment is faulty and social discrimination dubious. Still, during these first stages, many demented persons are capable of carrying on normal conversations and performing the ordinary physical feats of daily living.

B. *The moderate stages:* As time passes, what may be called a middle or moderate period of the disease sets in. Now moments of social noncommunication become increasingly common. The person will want to stay home most of the time and may abruptly sever old friendships, sometimes ending them in a tirade of accusations and ill will. Feelings previously kept in check are let out now, to the embarrassment of family and the deep chagrin of associates. Emotions become extremely unstable. Persons are no longer able to perform basic calculations; they may not be able to count, spell, or keep the thread of a story in mind. Sometimes at this point paranoia appears. One patient thought his grandchildren were spying on him whenever they came to visit. Another hid her valuable jewels throughout the house, causing no end of consternation when family members discovered diamond earrings in the coffee container and a jeweled wristwatch behind the toilet bowl.

Speech begins to slow in a noticeable way during the moderate period, as does verbal understanding. Persons may start repeating themselves or making repetitive sounds. One daughter of a stricken grandfather described it as the "ccccaaaacccccaaaa blues."

Catastrophic responses also mark this stage, with persons becoming suddenly irate over trifling incidents. Usually these reactions can be traced back to identifiable frustrations and to an inability to do what has heretofore been done with ease. For example, an elderly ex-printer's aide would fly into a dither whenever he washed his hands. At first his family thought the sound of the water was setting him off, but they soon discovered that he was reacting to the fact that he could no longer coordinate his fingers to lather the soap. At this stage persons also become socially inept. When talked at quickly or by more than one person at a time, they may react with withdrawal, anger, or even physical violence, poking or smacking the person who has confused them. Violent behavior, in fact, is sometimes quite prevalent among moderate-period dementia sufferers and must be given special attention (see Chapter 7).

During the moderate stage, persons are still more or less able to take care of their daily needs, but basic skills such as following a logical command or writing their name are diminished. *Apraxia,* the inability to perform skilled motor acts, may or may not manifest at this time. If it does, sick persons may stumble easily when getting up or may lean and sway while walking. They may have difficulty closing the lid of a jar, turning pages in a book, picking up small objects, or dialing the telephone.

C. *Severe stages:* In the later periods of dementia, sick persons can become prone to hallucinations (a delusion is a fixed, irrational idea, such as "The FBI is following me"; a hallucination is a false sensory perception, such as "Snakes are crawling about on the ceiling" or "Soldiers are attacking the apartment"). At this point persons become far more dependent on caregivers than ever before, yet simultaneously they become more abusive and unthankful too or, even worse, utterly cold and indifferent. Often they will not recognize the caregiver at all.

D. *Final stages:* In the final stages, patients lose almost all speech skills, all memory, and all intellectual abilities. They may also have difficulty walking, feeding themselves, and taking care of their toilet needs. They are incontinent now. They are confused. They recognize no one. They cannot remember things from moment to moment. They are gone.

Witnessing a loved relative in this last stage is one of the most heartbreaking experiences any family member can endure, but it is one that, mercifully, many demented patients and caregivers are spared. This is not because the disease ceases to progress during its later stages—progress continues to the end. It is because persons frequently die before they reach utter incapacitation. Nature is sometimes kind. In fact, it should be made clear that demented persons never actually die from the dementia itself; ironically, Alzheimer's is not technically a terminal illness. They die instead from the complications that attend the illness, such as heart failure, loss of appetite, and severe reduction of weight, or from the physical ravages of depression and from infections due to lowered resistance. Pneumonia, in fact, is probably the number one killer of AD patients. This ailment is not known as the "old person's friend" for nothing.

Finally, although no one is sure exactly how long a person will live from the onset of the disease to the end, an educated guess places the time span between four and seven years, plus or minus a few years on either end.

5. *Don't Get Upset Until It Happens*

This advice sounds directly contradictory to what was just said, but it isn't really. You owe yourself two debts as caregiver: one, to learn all you can about the disease and its expected symptoms, and two, to deal with these symptoms—and worry about them—only when they occur. Remember, the symptoms mentioned are by no means indigenous to every case of AD. Your loved one may experience all, some, or only a few. Moreover, these reactions tend to appear at certain times of day and not at others. It depends on how tired or anxious the person happens to be. For you, the most difficult task, perhaps, will be to balance anticipation of what to expect against your knowledge that with AD nothing is ever totally predictable.

Caregivers should thus remain as flexible as possible concerning the future. They should train themselves, as difficult as this process may be, not to worry about a particular problem until it arrives. Perhaps it never will.

> *Lawrence:* It never rains but it pours when you have a patient at home. You find yourself thinking, "What next?" and worrying about it. Thinking, "What's the next disaster? Will she lose her appetite? Will she start pissing on the couch? She's already ornery. More of the same, is that what I can expect?" Or worse than that. I've tended to make myself crazy guessing at what's around the corner. You asked me to give the best advice I could to other persons taking care of Alzheimer's patients. I'd say that they should try to take it one day at a time and not start fantasizing about things happening that aren't happening yet. Or may never happen.

So give yourself a break and take one day at a time.

6. Start Letting Go Early

Health professionals who work with the terminally ill often speak of something called "anticipatory grief." This term describes a process wherein caregivers start their grieving ahead of time, before their loved one has died or deteriorated beyond comprehensibility. The day the diagnosis is delivered is not too soon to begin this important inner work.

How does one grieve for a person not yet dead? There are several ways.

First, by squarely facing the fact that your loved one is suffering from a progressively degenerative disease and that the disease is irreversible.

Second, by realizing that spontaneous cures and reversals are extremely rare among demented patients.

Third, by accustoming yourself to the fact that soon ailing persons will lose their most vaunted cognitive faculties, their sympathy, their insight, their humor; slowly, invariably, these traits will vanish, one after the other, like leaves falling from a great tree.

Fourth, by sharing your pain and grieving problems with other caregivers in similar situations, preferably through groups sponsored by the Alzheimer's Disease and Related Disorders Association (ADRDA) or other self-help organizations (see Chapter 9).

Fifth, caregivers must understand that this sickness stems from actual disintegration of brain tissues, which means that yes, this person will die, perhaps in a few years' time. This is a most anguishing bullet to bite. But truth has a liberating effect as well as a sobering one. Operating from a realistic perspective allows caregivers to detour the silent embarrassments and sticky imbroglios that so often accompany denial. It allows them to assess their loved one's physical condition without illusions, to gauge how much quality time still remains, and to use this time wisely. It helps galvanize caregivers into locating resources, seeking needed financial and legal advice, setting up long-term care programs, and establishing relations with key health care professionals. Most important, by admitting to oneself at regular intervals that the loved one is sick and getting sicker and by giving oneself immunity to sorrow by, as it were, ingesting a small portion of sorrow every day, when the end actually arrives, caregivers will have already said most of their essential farewells.

7. *Make Use of Available Resources*

A number of resources are currently available to caregivers of AD sufferers—an amazingly large number, considering that Alzheimer's has been a major medical issue for less than twenty years. Certainly you owe it to yourself to learn about these valuable aids early in the game and to exploit them to the hilt.

What are these resources? First is the physician, of course. But behind this busy person stands a line of other strong shoulders on which you are invited to lean, and this group can help in apparent and not-so-obvious ways. They will naturally provide assistance around the house and with the sick person. But they will also support you in making important health care decisions, in gaining referrals and information, in relieving the daily caretaking burden, and in dealing with your own difficult states of mind. Key personnel include social workers, visiting nurses, homemakers and home health aides, nutritionists, occupational and speech therapists, psychologists and psychiatrists, and paid companions. Important too are the various professional agencies that help families cope with the day-to-day details of caregiving and the economic realities of home care. Among them are housekeeping, homemaker, and chore services; visiting nurse organizations; escort and transportation services; home health aid agencies; meal delivery services; information, consultation, and referral groups; and legal aid societies and local bar associations.

Finally, dozens of organizations, both profit and nonprofit, both community and private, feature departments that are set up exclusively to help families and caregivers of the handicapped elderly. A partial list includes adult day care centers, respite centers, senior centers, outpatient facilities and clinics, telephone reassurance services, personal emergency response systems, hospices, community mental health centers, and self-help and therapy groups for caregivers.

A recent national survey revealed that three quarters of persons saddled with the at-home custodial care of a demented person take care of their ward seven days a week without a break. Yet only 9.7 percent of these caregivers ever seek help from the services and organizations just listed. Indeed, there are many family members who insist on single-handedly shouldering all nursing responsibilities and who maintain that they alone are capable of satisfying the sick person's *real* needs. Believing that community services and professional home care agencies are costly window dressing at best, they will assure you that when all is said and done, the sick person's welfare depends exclusively on their own sweat and toil—even though these efforts may be carried out in an atmosphere of resentment, martyrdom, and exhaustion.

This is clearly a biased and self-defeating appraisal. Good home care personnel are highly experienced in the art of nurturing demented patients and are aware of therapeutic tricks and shortcuts that only people who have nursed a feeble elderly person can really know about. Usually these persons and services are affordable, and sometimes they come to caregivers free of charge via community services or governmental aid. Many caregivers, moreover, are older folks, people in their sixties and seventies for whom the strain of watching over a restive husband or a handicapped parent is especially severe. These caregivers will profit enormously from the wide range of public and commercial resources open to all. But they must learn that such aids are available in the first place, and in the second place, they must use them.

Outside aids definitely help. They relieve burdens caregivers once thought were unrelievable. They make life easier and saner. Try them and see. Above all, don't attempt to do it alone. Chapter 9 goes into this important subject in full detail.

8. Concentrate on Things You Can Do Right Now

Although there is little you can do to stem the oncoming tide of progressive dementia, there are plenty of practical, right-now tasks you can accomplish, both for yourself and for the sick person. A diagnosis of dementia invariably sets off a chain reaction at home, one that requires attention to the kinds of legal and accounting tasks that you and your family may never have given a second thought to before. Though these tasks may seem excruciating at first, they actually represent a kind of positive liberating force, simply because they entail matters that can be *controlled*, *altered*, and *improved*.

What matters are we speaking of? A sampling might include commissioning a lawyer knowledgeable in the field of aging; revising a patient's will; gaining power of attorney; setting up trusts and conservatorships; learning about insurance, veteran's benefits, and Medicare; looking into burial arrangements and prepaid funeral plans; establishing the logistics of long-term medical care; interviewing prospective home care agencies; establishing a representative payee to handle a patient's public benefits such as social security; appealing any denials for entitlements; and planning ahead for possible institutional care. All such activities have three elements in common:

1. They can be done today, right now, this very moment.
2. Doing them produces tangible, measurable results.
3. Once accomplished, they will supply you with a much needed feeling of achievement and control.

9. *Become Familiar with the Patient's Medications*

At the present time there are no actual medical treatments available for demented patients. Through the years various drugs have been touted as possible symptom relievers or even as cures, but none has been found that consistently slows down the degenerative neurological processes of dementia or stabilizes its symptoms. Recent advances with such drugs as L-dopa, however, demonstrate that it is possible to bring relief to forms of demential illnesses, in this case Parkinson's disease; and since the L-dopa miracle is based on subsidizing the brain's diminished supplies of the neurotransmitter dopamine, scientists are experimenting with several other neurotransmitters in hopes that a comparable medication for dementia will appear. While nothing concrete has yet emerged, many doctors are optimistic that breakthroughs will occur.

Have all dementia drugs proved equally ineffectual? Not exactly. Anecdotal stories abound concerning a number of home and professional remedies. For example, since it is believed that Alzheimer's stems from a deficit in the brain of the neurotransmitter acetylcholine, it was once hoped that heavy doses of the vitamin derivative choline would help. A wild rush to health food stores followed, and hopes were high. Some patients, it seems, reported improvement. A few even claimed to be cured. In the final tally, however, medical evidence determined that choline in its raw form is of no help whatsoever in the treatment of AD and that most of these wonder tales were unsubstantiated.

Other drugs that have been touted as having positive effects are the vasodilators, substances that produce dilation of the blood vessels (most popular are Cyclospasmol, Vasodilan, and Pavabid), and a medication called Hydergine, which is both a vasodilator and a metabolic enhancer.

Although physicians have mixed feelings about Hydergine (AD, some doctors reason, is not a vascular disease, so why use vasodilators to treat it?), it has apparently helped some patients *slightly*, apparently by increasing the flow of blood to their brains and hence *occasionally* improving mood and memory capacity. Test results have not been entirely negative in this regard, but the drug's helping capacities, if real, are relatively minor, and the substance certainly cannot be considered anything approaching a cure.

Among other drugs for Alzheimer's disease that have recently been tested are these:

- *Cholinergic agents:* choline, lecithin, and the agonists (RS 86, arecholine, and bethanechol)
- *Peptides:* vasopressin, ACTH 4-10, naloxone
- *Nootropic agents:* Pramiracetam, CI 911, Praxilene, Oxiracetam
- *Other general drugs:* chelating agents, Nimodipine, Vinpocetine

All are still in the experimental stages. Some have proved slightly beneficial but generally unsafe; others have tested as safe but not beneficial; and none has proved general effectiveness in helping demented persons get better. Thus if a medical professional one day informs you that drug X or drug Y or secret potion Z is of proven value for Alzheimer's disease and that taking it will help your relative in this way or that, walk quickly away. Such statements arise from ignorance or fraud. As yet we have no safe drugs that satisfactorily curb the symptoms of memory or speech loss in dementia or which reinstate the demented person's sense of logic and social awareness. Period.

What kind of drugs will demented persons most likely take, then? If they use drugs at all, they will probably use *psychotropics*, drugs that work on the mind and nervous system to palliate symptoms (specifically restlessness, violence, and anxiety) and which are designed to keep persons calm, relaxed, and sleeping well. The two general varieties of psychotropics are *tranquilizers* and *antidepressants.*

Tranquilizers: If the patient becomes especially restless, belligerent, or unable to sleep, tranquilizers (sometimes called *neuroleptics*) are used. Valium or Haldol, both old standbys, are often prescribed in these situations. Some tranquilizers are short-acting and keep patients sedated only for several hours. Others are long-acting, with effects that endure for days. Depending on the situation, your doctor will decide which variety is best.

Potential side effects of tranquilizers include dry mouth, blurred vision, drowsiness, and constipation. Occasionally so-called paradoxical reactions will result whereby the tranquilizer increases the symptoms it is designed to eliminate: Restless persons become more restless, sleepless persons become insomniacs. If a tranquilizer is prescribed, be sure your physician informs you ahead of time of its possible side effects and that he or she tells you what, if anything, you can do to relieve them.

Antidepressants: It is estimated that as many as twenty-five percent of demented patients are depressed. This condition can stem directly from the effects of the disease, or it may derive from secondary problems such as thyroid disorders or the effects of medication. Yet again, it may simply result from the dreary recognition on the part of the sick parties that they have chronic dementia and that their future is accordingly limited.

In cases of severe depression, physicians may prescribe antidepressants. These are designed to lift spirits and improve mood. The varieties likely to be prescribed include amitriptyline (brand names: Amitril, Endep, SK-Amitriptyline), desipramine (Norpramin, Pertofrane), doxepin (Adapin, Sinequan), imipramine (Antipress, Imavate, Presamine, SK-Pramine, Tofranil), nortriptyline (Aventyl, Pamelor), and trimipramine (Surmontil). Like tranquilizers, antidepressants produce a number of side effects including confusion, sedation, tremor, anxiety, and cardiac effects. Ask your doctor what to watch for and what to do if such effects occur.

Several other types of drugs may also be prescribed for the restless patient, including sedatives. When and if your doctor writes such prescriptions, be sure to ask what the drug is supposed to accomplish, what effects (and side effects) it produces, and how you can tell if it is working or not. AD patients tend to be highly sensitive to these medicines, and small dosages produce large effects. Most of the drugs mentioned also tend to stupefy patients and to reduce further the cognitive skills persons need to lead a quasi-normal life. As a physician once told one of our interviewed caregivers: "Why make an already confused, dazed person more confused and more dazed with drugs?"

Some doctors first advise caregivers to deal with problems via verbal and social tactics before resorting to medication. Dr. Robert Barrett, a neurologist in private practice and a specialist for many years in Alzheimer's disease, addresses the issue directly:

> There are not any medications today which you automatically prescribe for Alzheimer's disease. You can give a chemical straitjacket all right, a neuroleptic or something on that order. But it may cause more trouble than it's worth, what with side effects and making patients so drowsy during the day that you have to give them other medications to keep them awake during the day. It becomes a vicious cycle. Sedating persons so that they sleep all the day will reverse their sleeping patterns. They'll start staying up all night. Or they just lie around. That weakens their general state of health and makes them more vulnerable to disease. Not so great. I think twice and sometimes three times before I prescribe these drugs.

10. Develop a Long-Term Plan—and Use It

On hearing the diagnosis of AD, one of the most difficult emotions you will encounter is a sensation of bewildered inadequacy. An individual of great importance in your life is now ailing. Soon you will no longer be able to depend on this person to make you laugh or to serve you dinner, to drive you to work or to bring home a weekly paycheck, to oversee the thousand and one details of ordinary life that all of us take for granted when these jobs are in the hands of others.

The realization that a onetime partner and longtime sharer in life's panorama is becoming a helpless dependent creates feelings of panic and shock. "Who, ME? Deal with all that? Help!"

There is a wide selection of effective ways to cope with this frightening realization, and we will describe many of them in the chapters to come. Here, at the risk of repetition, let it be said again that one of the most efficient ways to come to terms with helplessness is to dwell on the things you can do now to make the situation more tolerable and manageable. Avoid the "can'ts" for the present. You will think about them later, perhaps. Now is the time to mobilize the "cans" and put them to constructive use. Emphasize your assets and your resources; stress planning and doing; go for action and involvement; deemphasize worry; put fear on hold.

The best way to realize this dynamic strategy is to look ahead. Ask yourself, What things will I have to know and do in the days and weeks to come? What problems will arise? What will I do about my finances, about social considerations, about learning nursing skills and dealing with family dynamics and hiring help and meeting with the doctor? How can I best prepare for all this? What steps can I take *right now?*

All caregivers are different, of course, and all have their own urgencies and objectives. At the same time, there are universal issues that arise when nursing a demented person that all of us must deal with, and this is where long-term preparation becomes critical. The chapters in Part II are organized around a number of these issues, with an emphasis on the hands-on, learn-it-yourself, do-it-now response to each. Taken together, this part of the book is meant to be a kind of guidebook, a dossier of specific health care instructions that will navigate you through the precarious waters ahead. The subjects addressed here center on the following issues and are all taken from information provided by Brookdale's professionals:

- *Making your household safe and secure for the sick person:* accident-proofing the house, avoiding floods and scalds, use of special equipment, etc.
- *Practical strategies for the patient's health maintenance and home care:* feeding, dressing, bathroom, hair care, sleep
- *Methods for ensuring your loved one's emotional well-being:* social life, recreation, dealing with stress and frustrations, therapeutic supports
- *Communicating with the demented person:* verbal and nonverbal ways of continuing to interact to the end
- *Methods of coping with abnormal behavior:* speech disruptions, aggressive behavior, restlessness, paranoia and delusions, verbal and physical abuse, etc.
- *Caregiver self-care:* emotional and physical supports to help maintain your own state of health
- *Collecting information on resources:* Using the best available organizations, professional services, self-help therapy, and community groups in your area
- *Financial contingencies:* Dealing with medical costs

In other words, most of the major issues and conflicts you are likely to face in the course of caregiving activities will be touched on in the chapters to follow, sometimes briefly, often in depth. It is suggested that you go through these sections carefully, collecting instructions that have special relevance to your needs, jotting down information that will be of practical help, and making note of all references that pertain to your specific situation.

For example, keep written records of any follow-up ideas you may have from your readings and of subjects you wish to learn more about. Outline project ideas. Make notes of your personal observations. Compile a bibliography of further reading. Write down lists, techniques, tricks, shortcuts, caveats, names and addresses, whatever you feel will be helpful and important. You will be glad to have these notes to refer to as time goes on.

Such a written sourcebook, based on your own experience and on information provided by professionals, serves as a tailor-made database to prepare you for the contingencies that arise during the course of home care. In this way you will plan your caregiving from a position of informed strength rather than out-of-control weakness. This is an extremely important goal to aim toward. Knowing where you want to go and what you must do to get there is a crucial end, both for maximizing your loved one's comfort and for taking care of your own inner needs. Remember, in the process of caregiving, planning will get you a quarter of the way to success, and knowledge another half. The last quarter then comes from your own special dedication, and from love. Onward and upward.

PART II

LONG-TERM
COPING PLAN

3

"Alzheimering" the Home: Making the Environment Safe, Efficient, and Peaceful

Caregiving for the Demented Person: What Is Really Necessary?

The goals of caretaking for a demented person can be spelled out in a few heartfelt words:

- Security
- Safety
- Freedom from physical pain
- Reduction of anxiety and frustration
- Loving nurturance and care

That's about it. There's not a great deal more we can do for demented persons other than help make them feel as loved, as comfortable, as stress-free as possible.

In this sense, however, the caregiver is off the hook. Once you get the hang of caregiving for an AD person, once you learn the person's habits and idiosyncrasies, there will be few curve balls. Set a regular schedule and stick to it: Predictable routine is extremely satisfying for the patient. And remember, AD caregiving has its own special satisfactions and rewards; do not think you are entering a one-way street. For some caregivers, the act of nursing an ailing AD person can become the most profound and meaningful experience of a lifetime.

The Caregiver Lives Here Too

Family members will want to start preparing for the domestic contingencies of caregiving right away. They will want to nip household safety hazards in the bud. They will want to make recreation and sleeping areas responsive to the sick person's physical requirements. They will want to arrange the furniture, the toilet facilities, the closets, the kitchen, and the bedroom so that the household works to serve medical and social needs. Nursing an Alzheimer's person begins and ends in the home.

At the same time—and this is an important reservation—family members will also want to maintain the sanctity of their own living quarters, so that they will not come to feel resentful or intruded on by the ailing person's demanding presence. The rest of this chapter will deal with a number of important ways in which the balance between medical needs and domestic peace of mind can be maintained. It will explain techniques caregivers can use to make their private dwelling a safe, happy space for the patient and at the same time maintain it as a congenial and manageable place for their own needs as well.

Adapt, Don't Change

The moment it becomes apparent that a spouse or relative is suffering from dementia, caregivers are often gripped by the impulse to *do something*, anything, simply to gain a feeling of control over an out-of-control situation. Since the nearest manageable thing is one's environment, we frequently see family members at this stage frantically buying new furniture and hammering up partitions.

Such haste can make waste. It can be a mistake, first of all, because the caregiver lives here too and has territorial rights: To make drastic household changes right away without carefully assessing the sick person's actual needs will only cause anger for everyone plus a lot of unnecessary work.

It is a mistake too for a more fundamental reason. The AD victim, especially in the early stages when he or she is still in command of many mental faculties, desperately needs to be surrounded by a predictable, familiar setting. To build in bureaus and replace beds may be an intelligent plan from the standpoint of administrative efficiency, but on the human side it can be a deeply disturbing threat to the patient's self-image and all-important status quo. It may make enormous logistic sense to move grandmother out of her long-established upstairs lodgings down to a first-floor bedroom where her shaky legs will no longer have to negotiate the winding stairs. But from Grandmother's point of view, her already failing abilities to recognize landmarks when moving from room to room will receive an additional insult from this confusing change in setting. Here the best of intentions quickly makes a bad situation worse.

You get the point. Demented individuals struggle desperately and pathetically to remember things that normal persons take for granted: "This is a dining room chair. I sit on it when I eat. This is a coat hanger. I hang my shirt on it at night." So goes the inner litany as the person struggles to get around.

What then is the best way of arranging the AD household without causing wide-scale disruption? According to several health care professionals associated with the Brookdale Center, there are four rules of thumb to follow:

1. Adapt the home; don't change it entirely.
2. Simplify the home; don't strip it bare.
3. Modify the environment to the person's particular needs—and do no more.
4. Balance your own needs against those of the AD person—and strike a happy medium between the two.

Let's go over in detail how these tasks can be best followed, taking each important living area of your house or apartment as examples.

"Alzheimering," Room by Room

The Bedroom

Beds.   Most public health nurses do *not* recommend that families with a demented person at home immediately rent a hospital bed. For one thing, the ailing person's bed and mattress constitute a highly charged security object; to suddenly replace it with a looming metallic apparatus may produce sleep problems and disruption anxieties. Such objects will also remind persons of the hospital itself and hence of sickness and helplessness, an anxiety-provoking set of associations to say the least. In addition, regular-sized beds are lower to the ground than hospital beds and offer better ease of access. Negotiating the covers can also become a confusing ordeal, and many accidents occur among the demented in the critical morning and evening hours when getting in and out of bed. (It is not unusual to hear of demented persons who have tangled themselves up in a blanket and gone catapulting to the floor, breaking a hip or leg in the process.) The hospital-style bed, with its puzzling side rails and electric cables, multiplies the chances of such accidents, and its extra height from the floor increases the possibilities of a fracture should the person take a fall.

Eventually, however, when the person becomes permanently bed-bound, a hospital bed will probably be needed. When this time arrives, a flotation mattress is considered the best resting surface, both because of its comfort and because it reduces the incidence of bedsores (more on this later). If you do import a hospital bed into your home, position it in a corner of the room so that the person is prevented from falling (or climbing) out of bed by two wall surfaces.

Harmful Objects.   Remove all sharp, heavy, and breakable objects such as pencils, typewriters, tools, glass objects, plus small knickknacks that can be popped into the mouth. But leave the furniture in place unless it presents an obvious safety hazard (pointed corners, barbed handles, chairs that rock, folding tables and drawers that pinch fingers). Likewise, empty the shelves of items that stab, stick, or cut. Chairs and sofas in general are most useful to demented persons when they have wide armrests and high backs to facilitate easy rising. Steam radiators and exposed hot surfaces should be covered with insulating material or barricaded off by pieces of furniture. Keep chairs away from all electric and steam heaters: Patients have been known to rest an arm or leg absent-mindedly on a radiator while dozing and to be severely burned.

Rugs.   Scatter rugs offer potential slippage problems and should be well tacked down. Carpeting is a better alternative for several reasons: It cuts noise, it prevents slipping, and it breaks the surface impact in case of falls. It is also cozy and attractive as far as the caregiver is concerned.

Lamps and Light Sources.   Be sure all lamp and extension cords are positioned out of the line of walking traffic. Overhead ceiling fixtures offer the best lighting for a person's room. Next in rank come fixtures that can be fastened directly to walls. Bedside lamps are easily knocked off, the hot bulbs of floor lamps will burn unwary fingers, and trailing electric cords can be a hazard to everyone. Install several night lights in the person's room near bathroom entrances and by main doorways.

Wall Hangings.   Keep all wall hangings, framed pictures, and photographs in place unless they are disturbing to the sick person (one elderly demented woman started to tear her shirt every time she saw a picture of her former flower garden). In general, persons enjoy looking at pretty, cheerful pictures, especially those that carry positive associations: photos of family and friends, an ancestral home, or a familiar landscape. One Hungarian grandmother became especially calm and enthusiastic when family members showed her a framed tintype of the street in Budapest where she and her husband had been married sixty years before. The person may not recognize exactly what the pictures show, but the images are somehow reminiscent of better times.

Cues.   One of the practical techniques for helping a demented person remain comfortable at home is the use of cues. Cues are visual or auditory reminders, memory joggers that individuals in the early stages of AD can use to help them remember what's what. A typical cue may be a sign on the closet door saying "Clothes Closet" or a picture of a toilet on the bathroom door. A more creative cue might be a tape recording on a clock-radio/tape recorder programmed to go off at a certain time of day with instructions for dressing or for taking medication.

Cues are particularly useful in the bedroom. Since the person may not remember from day to day where her dresses are kept or in which part of the room her blouses are stored, you can help by taking a photograph (or drawing a picture) of a dress, a blouse, or a shoe, and pasting it over the appropriate closet or drawer. If the room has several closets and each has a separate door, this method will be particularly useful (some caregivers remove the closet doors entirely to provide easier access). In one household where a demented parent's room had several closet doors, family members helped the person tell them apart by painting the bathroom door a deep red, the hall door a light green, the closet doors blue, and so forth. Don't minimize the value of such cues—they work.

Quick Checklist for Bedroom Safety

All hot surfaces such as light bulbs and radiators are pro-   _____
tected.
All small objects that can go into the mouth are removed.   _____
Loose rugs are either secured to the floor with tacks or   _____
double-sided tape, or are permanently removed.
All sharp surfaces and sharp objects are placed out of the   _____
person's reach.
Sofas, chairs, and beds are not too high off the ground.   _____
Lighting is ample, without dangerous electric cords or   _____
lamps nearby that can be knocked over.

The Bathroom

Poisonous Substances.   More accidents happen to older persons in bathrooms than in any other part of the house, and this statistic includes the demented population as well. Bathroom safety must be considered from several standpoints. First, poisonous substances. Remove all detergents, bleaches, ammonia, and toxic cleaning products and store them far from the person's reach. Ditto razors, scissors, and sharp pointed objects. Many demented persons lose judgment early on concerning what can and cannot go into their mouths, and brightly colored pills and capsules are a real temptation. Confine all medications and poisonous cleaning substances to their own drawer or closet, and keep it locked if possible. Locks on the bathroom door should open from the outside as well as the inside.

Ambulatory Safety.   All electrical appliances should be taken out of the bathroom immediately and all extension cords and dubious electrical wires removed. Bathroom lighti is best when controlled via a switch by the door. *Never* leave a table lamp or plug-in radio in the bathroom. Handrails and grab bars fastened securely to the walls near the bath and toilet will provide much-needed support and will discourage persons from grabbing a towel bar or shower curtain for lack of anything better to hold on to should they slip. If possible, select a grab bar that is conspicuously and contrastingly colored for rapid identification. (Grab bars can be purchased from several health supply dealers. See "Useful Equipment" toward the end of this chapter.)

Baths.   If either the bath or sink is drained by a lever plug, it's a good idea to remove the entire plug unit—the units usually slip in and out on their own—and replace them with old-fashioned rubber stoppers. In this way drainage problems can be more easily controlled, and intact patients will be able to manipulate these rubber plugs on their own when bath time is over. Never fill a tub higher than one quarter capacity. Tub or shower chairs (with secure backrests and legs with rubber tips) are excellent aids for elderly persons who are shaky on their feet.

Toilet.   Falls while on the toilet are common and should be carefully monitored. A grab bar installed next to the toilet seat will help persons sit and stand when using the facilities. Adjustable commodes and low toilets are available from plumbing supply houses. Always use hard toilet seats. The cushioned varieties are slippery and can contribute to falls.

Slippery Surfaces.   Place nonskid tape over all slippery surfaces, especially in the bathtub and shower, and use liquid soap instead of soap bars to prevent slipping. Nonslip bath mats or wall-to-wall bathroom carpeting are also useful if the floor is tiled and slippery. In the Johnsons' household the family keeps several thick pieces of bathroom rug on reserve to place on the floor after Grandmother has taken her splashy shower. The rug absorbs the water and provides a nonslip surface for Grandmother to walk on.

Scald Prevention.   Demented persons in moderate to advanced stages tend to lose their discrimination between hot and cold, and scalds frequently occur. There are several mechanical methods for preventing such accidents. First, turn the thermostat on your hot water heater down low. Hot water heaters are accessible in most houses and apartments, and temperature control is a simple matter of turning a knob. If you don't feel confident making this adjustment yourself, consult a handyman or a plumber. City apartments sometimes have a hot water thermostat for each apartment.

Second, in the person's bathroom, the knobs on the faucets and showers can easily be taken off with screwdriver and pliers and stored in a safe place. This simple act will save you a lot of worry and will put bathroom control entirely in your hands. When patients need to bathe, you retrieve the handles, turn on the water, set the temperature, and leave them to their pleasure. Hot water in the sink can be shut off by turning the left shut-off knob below the drain spout. Many patients prefer to use hand-held shower heads rather than those fixed to the wall. These can be purchased at any hardware store and are relatively simple to install.

Quick Checklist for Bathroom Safety

All medications and toxic substances have been removed   _____
and put in a safe place.

Grab bars have been installed, nonslip tape has been ap-   _____
plied, and general slip prevention measures have been
taken.

Antiscald measures such as removing faucet handles and   _____
turning down water temperature have been taken.

The Kitchen

Second to the bathroom in hazard potential is the kitchen, repository of scalding liquids, unattended flames, slippery floors, hot pans, and toxic cleansers. Begin by placing all knives and sharp objects out of sight. Install childproof door latches on any cabinets that contain breakable objects or household cleaning chemicals. Follow this up by keeping your glasses, silverware, china, kitchen tools and small appliances, and the like in a protected area away from easy reach. However, by no means get rid of your important kitchen utensils. You have the right to own them and to use them. Simply put them out of harm's way. A few hours spent rearranging drawers, cabinets, and shelves is usually all that's needed.

High on the danger list is the heat generated by stove burners, be they gas or electric. Accustomed to cooking for himself in his large kitchen apartment, Donald G. got into trouble in the days before his condition was diagnosed when he placed several English muffins in an electric toaster oven and promptly fell asleep. The toaster remained on for more than an hour and eventually heated up so much that it ignited a nearby roll of plastic wrap. Fortunately, Donald woke up a minute or two after the fire had broken out, smelled smoke, and ran to the kitchen. By the time he arrived a good portion of the walls and cabinets had already been scorched, and it took several frightening minutes to extinguish the flame. The next week he did exactly the same thing.

What to do about such potentially disastrous situations? Perhaps the quickest solution is to remove the knobs from the kitchen stove and to keep them in a safe place when the stove is off. This is a major inconvenience but a guaranteed problem solver. Another alternative is to lock the kitchen door. If this is not feasible, an accordian gate across the entrance to the kitchen secured with a small lock will serve the same end. It is wise not to allow the patient into the kitchen without supervision.

Persons with gas stoves can thwart fire potential by having a shut-off valve attached to their incoming gas line. The valve is then kept in the off position when not in use. Utility companies, depending on their regional policy, will sometimes provide families of demented persons with valve installation free of charge or for a very low fee, but only if you can offer medical proof that an AD patient resides in your home. Yet another alternative, perhaps the best of the lot, is to use tamperproof stove knobs, which can be purchased wherever childproofing equipment is sold. Tamperproof water faucets are also available, a real boon for those who have had an ailing relative turn on the tap for a drink of water, then forget to shut it off and walk away, leaving the water to run—and run, and run.

Demented patients, like children, are often attracted to the glittering reds, yellows, and greens featured on commercial packaging. Since many cleaning products come in vivid wrappings, it is best to lock up all soap powders, detergents, chemicals, drain cleaners, polishes, and waxes inside a cabinet and store the key out of sight nearby. As long as the key is hidden, chances are the patient will not remember where you keep it.

Watch out for small "eatable" kitchen items such as matches, tooth-picks, pencil stubs, plastic sandwich bags, wrappers, and strong spices such as pepper, cloves, and especially whole nutmegs (only one of these powerful little nuts needs to be ingested to produce delirium and hallu-cinations). Are any jagged edges exposed? Are sharp corners in evi-dence? If so, rubber cornerpieces can be fit over all jutting surfaces. Polyurethane sealers on floors offer a more permanent shiny surface than waxes and are a good deal less slippery.

Patients in the early stages of dementia who can still use the kitchen without heavy supervision will have a difficult time manipulating kitchen machinery or performing relatively complex maneuvers such as unscrew-ing a jar or buttering a piece of bread. Homemade inventions help in this area; for example:

- A square block of wood bolted to the lid of a jar will afford a firm turning grip.
- A twelve-by-twelve-inch wooden board with two dowels nailed on one surface to form a right angle will serve as a caddy to hold objects in place: bread for buttering, packages to be unwrapped, bowls to be stirred.
- Double-sided suction cups keep the bottom of bottles or mixing bowls firmly fixed to counter surfaces.
- Nonslip cutting boards can be made by hammering several rows of 1¼-inch galvanized nails into an inch-thick board (so that just the tips of the nails come through on the other side) and securing the reverse side to the work surface by means of double-sided suction cups. The protruding nails on the exposed side of the board, their tips flattened a bit for safety by a blow or two from a hammer, will then hold vegetables in place while they are being peeled or sectioned. Note that unlike AD patients, MID sufferers some-times have the ability to learn how to use simple machines and to retain these memories from day to day. For them, adapted kitchen appliances and machinery will be especially useful.

Commercially speaking, lid top turners, available at any hardware store, will eliminate the frustration of difficult jar and bottle top removal. Perforated metal tea-infusing spoons can be used to stir tea as well as to brew it; they are easier and quicker than standard tea bags. An inch-thick piece of foam rubber placed in the sink under the plate drainer or near kitchen working surfaces will discourage breakage. Nonslip rubber mats on the floor will prevent falling, especially when floors are wet. Check the items featured at the end of this chapter for further suggestions on commercial around-the-house home care equipment.

Quick Checklist for Kitchen Safety

All kitchen machinery, breakables, sharp surfaces, and po-   _____
tentially dangerous objects are stored in a safe place.

Adequate stove safety and flame control have been   _____
established.

All household cleaners and chemicals have been stored in a   _____
safe, out-of-reach location.

All small objects that can be put into the mouth have been   _____
removed.

All slippery floor surfaces are covered or protected.   _____

Stairs

With its ever-present potential for slips, trips, and tumbles, stair-cases are responsible for almost a quarter of all falling accidents that occur in the homes of the elderly.

For starters, remember that uncovered stairs are slippery stairs, especially if the nosing on the edge of the tread is rounded. Nonslip tape, rubber treads, or strip carpeting secured to all exposed surfaces will reduce this potential hazard severalfold. Just be sure your carpeting is well secured and meticulously tacked down. Loose rugs make the stair-case area an instant danger zone.

All staircases should be equipped with a solidly supported banister, and nonskid tape is sometimes wrapped around banisters to increase their grip security. Some families install a second banister or extra grab rail on the opposite wall of the staircase to provide double insurance. However, going up and down stairs with both arms extended puts the patient in an awkward position, and some experts think that one well-installed railing does the job better than two.

The brighter the lighting in a stairway, the better. Keep a light on twenty-four hours a day in this area if possible. An extension gate placed at the top of the stairs will prevent tumbles; a gate at the bottom will discourage patients from using the stairs when no one is watching.

If a fall does occur, chances are it will cause less harm if all sharp, jutting objects (such as tables, chairs, or umbrella stands) are removed from the bottom of the stairway. Some caregivers arrange extra padding at the foot of the stairs, just in case. Be careful to lock all cellar and attic doors: A dive onto cement or down winding stairs will be a good deal more bone-shattering than a short tumble onto carpeted steps. Since AD sufferers frequently dawdle when using the stairs, losing their concentration and then forgetting entirely where they are headed, caregivers sometimes paint large arrows on the walls as a reminder to patients that they are *going somewhere*.

Banister-style elevators are available and can be installed on most staircases, usually with minimal damage to walls and woodwork. No special wiring is required for these rigs (most stairway lifts plug into a 110-volt outlet), and the track on which the seat runs is no more than a foot wide. Still, there are drawbacks. Stairway elevators are expensive, costing $2000 or more *before* installation. At moderate and advanced levels of dementia, the patient will no longer be able to operate these machines alone, and the caregiver will have to do all the work, placing the patient on the seat, strapping him in, taking him off again at the top. However, if you can afford it, and if stairs are a major problem in your home, a stairway elevator may be worth looking into. Check the listings at the end of this chapter for more information.

Quick Checklist for Staircase Safety

All slippery staircase surfaces are covered.   _____

All staircase rugs are well secured.   _____

All sharp corners near the stairs are covered or removed.   _____

A strong banister is installed on all staircases.   _____

The doors to basement and attic stairs are kept closed and   _____
    locked.

Staircase lighting is adequate and kept on twenty-four hours   _____
    a day.

Protective gates are installed at staircase tops and bottoms.   _____

Other Concerns

Access.   Make certain that all access paths to different rooms in the house or apartment are kept clear. For instance, if the person is in a wheelchair, be sure that the path between the bathroom and the living room is unobstructed. If the person is walking-impaired, be sure that routes through hallways, foyers, and walk-in porches are not blocked with bulky furniture. If the person has a recurrent problem running into furniture or tripping on a step-down, pieces of reflector tape strategically placed will serve as warnings.

Electrical Cords.   Place all electrical cords out of reach. Cover exposed wall sockets with two-pronged plastic socket protectors, available at most hardware and variety stores. Beware of "octopus" plugs and overhanging wires that can be pulled out or ripped down. Watch out for table appliances, radios, clocks, and lamps with cords—these can be tripped over or pulled violently to the floor.

Locks.   If nocturnal wandering is a problem, you may wish to install locks with external keyways, so that patients can be locked into their rooms at night. Tumble bolts are more difficult to manipulate than regular button locks and are recommended for all AD households.

If patients are in the habit of tampering with locks and undoing them, install a second lock on the same door that turns in a different direction from the first; for example, if the top bolt turns clockwise, have the bottom bolt turn counterclockwise. This little trick will confuse patients and discourage them from opening practically any door.

An ever-looming problem, of course, is that patients will lock themselves in and then not be able to figure out how to reverse the process. This occurs frequently in bathrooms and lock-up closets. A demented elderly plumber named Ronnie once maneuvered himself into the basement, locked the door behind him, and proceeded to get into his son's household paints. By the time the family removed the door and removed Ronnie, he had already swallowed several varieties of oil paint and had to be rushed to the hospital. This unfortunate scenario could have been prevented with the proper use of locks.

One way around lock-in problems is simply to remove all inside locks from all inside doors and replace them with hook-and-eye locks. Hook-and-eyes are difficult for most demented patients to figure out, and if the locks do by chance get latched from the inside, they can easily be forced open without having to break down the door. Another solution is to secure a piece of tape across the face of the lock so that the bolts are prevented from engaging. Note also that some patients enjoy grabbing hold of doorknobs and rattling them for hours at night. If this is a problem in your home, replace the old knob with a new, single-unit knob that does not rattle.

The Yard.   A primary danger here is the swimming pool. Statistics on the number of AD patients who have drowned in backyard pools are not available, but according to the reckoning of several experts, pool drownings are the number-one cause of backyard deaths among the homebound demented. If you do have a pool, keep it covered in the winter and highly supervised in the warm weather months. If there is a pool in the neighborhood, alert the pool's owner that you have an Alzheimer's patient living in your home.

Demented persons should be carefully watched when out-of-doors. On the slightest provocation, they will put sticks or rocks into their mouths, trip on roots or weeds, miss their balance, hit their heads, lose their way. While fresh air is certainly an important health asset, a porch or an enclosed area is the best place to get it. Also, make sure that all front and back walkways leading up to your house are even and that there are no roots, broken cobblestones, jutting bricks, or uneven gravel surfaces to cause trips and falls. If front door stairs tend to be wet and slippery at certain times of the year, rubber runners can be placed on the treads. These sometimes come in different colors, a boon to visibility for everyone.

The Car.   Car safety is much the same for the demented person as it might be for any passenger. Seat belts are critical, not only because they protect the occupant in an accident but also because they discourage moving about in the car. More important still, non-seat-belted AD passengers are unpredictable and potentially dangerous to everyone in the car. They may suddenly snatch at the driver's arm, reach for the steering wheel, or try to tamper with the controls. Forewarned is forearmed. The backseat is ordinarily better suited than the front for transporting demented passengers, though again, be sure the person is wearing a seat belt. Patients may otherwise be tempted to climb into the front seat while the car is in motion or to grab the driver from behind.

Pick up and put away any small articles left around the automobile interior. These can be popped into the mouth in seconds. The glove compartment should be locked, and all stray items like pencils, cigarette stubs, coins, and mirror ornaments are best kept out of sight. Many autos now come equipped with special backseat child locks that can only be opened from the outside. These devices are excellent for your needs. If the person tends to tamper with car door hardware, heavy-duty tape stretched over all vulnerable knobs, handles, and buttons will prevent accidents.

A special problem some caregivers confront is the demented person's fear of entering motor vehicles, especially the large vans frequently used to transport persons to day care centers or respite programs. Although there is not always a great deal that can be done to talk loved ones out of these phobias—"No one in the world can be more stubborn than an Alzheimer's patient who has it in his mind not to do a thing," the wife of an AD patient remarked—the one trick that has been used with some success is to have the rider *back into the vehicle.* If persons are not looking directly at the car while entering it, they often have less fear and will sometimes allow themselves to be loaded without protest.

Planning for a Wheelchair in the Home.   If the patient is wheel-chairbound, certain adjustments in the home will facilitate efficient movement from room to room. Here are a few dos and don'ts for intelligent wheelchair planning:

● Do get a chair that is light, is relatively transportable, and which folds up into a convenient size. A standard wheelchair with footrest weighs around thirty-five pounds, a narrow one around thirty. Anything much heavier will not be practical if you move the patient frequently. If the chair is to be used only occasionally, it is probably OK to buy a model "off the rack." For heavy use, however, which will someday become a reality for most demented persons, have a physical therapist suggest a chair size that is properly suited to the sitter's body size and weight. If you buy a chair directly from a health equipment dealer, such organizations sometimes have specialists on hand who can help customize the wheelchair to the patient's needs.

● Do have a special location in the home where you can store the wheelchair when it is not in use. Possible places include foyers, halls, laundry rooms, walk-in closets, pantries, apartment hallways, under a staircase, or in a vestibule.

● Do lay down roll-out rubber mats over all the floor and rug areas that you want to protect. Constant wheelchair use will scuff and abrade almost any floor surface.

● Do check the height of all sofas and sitting places in your home to be certain that the person can transfer from wheelchair to seat with relative ease. Ideally, the height of the wheelchair and the chair or sofa should be the same.

● Do use ramps to simplify the process of pushing a wheelchair up entranceway stairs or onto step-up areas. Ramps can be purchased from suppliers of home health equipment (see "Useful Equipment" toward the end of this chapter) or homemade out of plywood. Some caregivers purchase metal motorcycle ramps from local auto supply dealers. These consist of two parallel lengths that are placed beneath the wheels and can be carried from room to room with relative ease.

• Do plan out access routes throughout the house, and do arrange all furniture to accommodate these routes.

• Do have a place near the patient's bed where he or she can get in and out of the chair with ease. Do surround this area with soft rugs in case of a fall.

• Do make sure the distance from the open bathroom door to the toilet is sufficient to allow the wheelchair full entry into and use of the bathroom. Note that bathroom doors are often the narrowest doors in the house. Before purchasing a wheelchair, make certain that it can pass into the bathroom. It may be necessary to remove the door and replace it with an accordion door or even a curtain.

• Do make provisions for securing persons into the wheelchair with belts or straps whenever you take them out-of-doors (demented wheelchair-bound patients have been known to climb out of their chairs in public places when the caregiver is not looking, occasionally with drastic results).

• Don't leave the wheelchair in places around the house where you can bump into it or fall over it at night.

• Don't leave the footplates on the chair when it is not in use. Your shins, and everyone else's, will thank you.

• Don't purchase a wheelchair until you have measured the width of all household doorways. Standard wheelchairs measure 24½ inches across and have an 18-inch seat. Sometimes they come in wider sizes, sometimes in smaller. Check first.

• Don't purchase a wheelchair until you are confident of its turning capacities. If the chair is going to be pushed around a small apartment or a house with many rooms, it will have to negotiate some sharp pivots. Measure its turning circumference first before renting or purchasing.

• Don't let wheelchair routes run too close to fine furniture or breakable objects. Occupants may run into or grab at these items as they go by.

• Don't load the person into the chair while on a slick surface. Even the most competent caregivers can lose their grip—and their footing—under slippery conditions.

A Caregiver's Household Rights: Maintaining
Your Own Space

In the midst of all these caregiver requirements, do not neglect your own sense of home and private space, and do not allow the sick person's domestic needs to totally usurp your own. This is easier said than done, perhaps, in the midst of so many patient-oriented demands. Still, there are bottom-line measures that can be taken to help neutralize these feelings of being taken over and surrounded. Try not to neglect them. They have real value as far as your own survival is concerned. A few of the most significant ones follow.

• Have at least one room or area of the home that is exclusively yours, off-limits to the patient. Keep it sacrosanct, an oasis of quiet and repose. This area can be a bedroom, a rumpus room, even a porch or a made-over basement. One interviewed caregiver fixed up an attached garage and went to it from time to time to smoke and contemplate. June R., a twin who stayed home in her family house in Maine to nurse her Alzheimer's sister, described this protected locale as her "quiet place":

> Whenever I feel like I'm going to scream or blow my stack or punch [sister] Louise in the teeth, I head for my quiet place. I sit there and count to a hundred if necessary, then I take some deep breaths and look out the window at the bay for a couple of minutes. It's calming, and Louise can't follow me in here. The qualifications for my quiet space are that, one, it be comfortable; two, it be off-limits to my sister; and three, it afford me short and pleasurable little minivacations from life.

• Furnish your quiet area with things you enjoy, such as good books, magazines, games, a TV, or sound equipment. Keep objects in this area that are particularly valuable to you or that the patient could conceivably break or hide.

• Have a lock on the door of your private space that you can close whenever you wish. Honor your own territorial imperative.

• Keep a strongbox for storing money and valuables. Jewels, coins, stamps, and any other bright or colorful objects will attract demented patients. Since somewhere in the recesses of their minds many of them recall that these objects have value, they may end up hiding your wallet, stuffing dollar bills into old books, or throwing jewels down the drain. Margaret L. came home one night to discover that her husband, Lucian, an AD sufferer, had pried into her personal files. He had removed several sheaves of stocks and bonds and was busily tearing them into neat shreds and stuffing them under the desk blotter. The next day Margaret removed all her valuable papers and placed them in a safe-deposit box at the bank.

Useful Equipment for "Alzheimering" the Home

Although home health supplies such as grooming equipment, pans and urinals, standing aids, exercise equipment, reachers, and safety rails are of use to demented persons only in the early stages when they are still ambulatory and in command of some cognitive faculties, these aids often remain valuable to the caregiver up to very end. Indeed, we live in the era of a home care equipment boom, and it would be a shame not to reap its benefits. Health supplies can be purchased directly from mail order dealers, from an increasingly large number of drugstores, from orthopedic suppliers, or directly from hospitals. (At one time the primary customers for medical equipment, hospitals have recently become entrepreneurs in the field of home health supplies themselves.) Even some major retail stores offer weighty catalogs featuring home health care goods, and several of these companies such as Sears and Montgomery Ward maintain in-store departments where a sometimes bewildering variety of equipment is kept on display.

With so many vendors, buying can become a confounding affair. To cut through the complexities, ask yourself basic questions about your home care needs:

- What do my doctor and the other health care professionals think I need in the way of home care equipment?
- What health supply items are really necessary? Which ones will quickly become obsolete? What are my priorities?
- How do prices compare between vendors? If the incontinence pads or the wheelchairs sold by one dealer are a lot cheaper than those sold by another company, perhaps the quality is a lot lower too. Examine all bargains before committing yourself.
- What about warranties and guarantees? Will the vendor replace defective items, or must I go to the trouble of sending goods back to the manufacturer?
- What organizations can I contact to get objective information about the quality of home care equipment?

In answer to the last question, there are two principal sources that educate caregivers concerning home health care equipment. First is

Abledata, a service of the National Rehabilitation Information Center (NARIC) in Washington (4407 Eighth Street NE, Washington, DC 20017; 800-346-2742, 301-588-9284). NARIC provides a comprehensive search and evaluation service for over ten thousand home health care products. They charge a small fee for the search. List your needs, then get in touch with them directly for the particulars.

The Accent on Information System (P.O. Box 700, Bloomington, IL 61701; 309-378-2961), an affiliate of *Accent on Living*, a magazine for the disabled, will search the data bank of a major state college to help you find information on your specific in-home requirements.

As far as actual home care equipment goes, some caregivers are not fully aware of the remarkably wide variety of do-it-yourself health care gadgets that are presently available by mail. The following list, geared especially to the demented patient, is only a brief sampling of what is presently on the market. Addresses of suppliers are provided at the end of this section.

Home Care Equipment Sampler for the Caregiver

Easiturn Faucet Handles.   Rigid plastic handles seven inches long that attach to faucet knobs and make turning water on and off easier for movement-impaired persons. This device comes in handy in the early stages of dementia when a person can still perform many ordinary household tasks. (Abbey Medical)

Security Light.   Emergency light turns itself on automatically whenever a power outage occurs; it is practically essential in any home that houses an invalid, especially in areas where blackouts are common. (Arthritis Self Help Products)

Incontinence Pants and Underpads.   All varieties for all needs and situations. (HSA Health Supplies of America)

Grab Bars.   An assortment for tubs, toilets, halls. (Cleo, Inc.)

One-Touch Blood Pressure Monitor.   Lets you take a patient's vital signs without using a blood pressure cuff. The device slips onto the patient's finger and provides a quick digital readout. (Medical Self-Care)

Pill Organizer.   The Mediplanner pill organizer dispenses exact dosages. Twenty-four compartments marked with big letters (and in braille) hold a full week's worth of medication. (HSA Health Supplies of America)

Round-the-Clock Multiple Time Switch.   The James Remind-O-Timer starts or stops household appliances at whatever time of day you program it for. Can be used to turn radios, air conditioners, lights, alarms, and other appliances on and off automatically. (American Foundation for the Blind)

One-Way Intercom.   You can hear, but no one can hear you. Used primarily to keep tabs on newborns and infants, this intercom is also useful for keeping an ear on the elderly demented. Can be purchased from any electronic appliance store.

Triangular Suction Plate.   Three suction cups are positioned on the outer edge of the plate to prevent it from moving while the patient eats. Other useful eating utensils for movement-impaired patients include the high-sided dish, the no-tip glass, the wheelchair beverage holder and cup holder with cup, the no-tip snorkel lid mug, the convalescent no-dribble feeding cup, and disposable bibs. (Fred Sammons, Inc.)

Hardwood Bedside Chair with Hidden Toilet.   A toilet seat cleverly concealed in a comfortable and decorative wooden chair, suitable for use in the living room or bedroom. A fine way to reduce the socially aware patient's embarrassment over having a commode nearby and in plain sight.

Flotation Bed Pan.   Synthetic sheepskin–covered pad rolls out and helps protect and cushion the entire trunk and back of a bedbound person. Requires no leveling pad. (Spenco Medical Corp.)

Lateral Trunk Support.   Foam-padded curved plastic support designed to bolster the individual who is unable to stand erect due to muscle weakness or imbalance. Also available are torso supports and trunk support safety vests. (Fred Sammons, Inc.)

Handi-Trak Economy Wheelchair Ramp.   The two tracks that make up this piece of equipment are portable, fit into a car, and can be easily moved from room to room by a single person. (Cleo, Inc.)

Dental Emergency Kit.   Designed by a dentist to provide temporary relief from common dental problems. Kit comes with step-by-step, color-coded instructions. Great to keep elderly patients' frequent dental problems under control. (Carolina Health and Fitness)

Talking Clock.   For patients obsessed with knowing the time, this pocket-sized talking clock recites the time on command. It also has an alarm and a radio. (American Foundation for the Blind)

In-Bed Shampoo Tray.   For washing a bedridden patient's hair. (Cleo, Inc.)

Cervical Pillow.   Designed by an orthopedic surgeon, it promotes restful sleep for persons with neck problems. Packed with polyester fiber, it is machine washable and dryable. (Medical Self Care)

Electric Self-feeder.   Feeds the patient who is no longer able to use his or her arms. Spoon automatically moves toward the mouth. Sometimes useful in the last stages of dementia. (Fred Sammons, Inc.)

Suction Holders.   Double-sided suction cups are used to anchor dishes, glasses, bowls, and other items to the table. (Fred Sammons, Inc.)

Toilet Safety Armrest.   Helps persons steady themselves while using the privy. (Cleo, Inc.)

Hydraulic Patient Lift.   Large power lift provides a safe mechanical means for transporting the patient (in a sling chair) from one area of the room to another. Expensive, elaborate, large, but sometimes needed. (Abbey Medical)

Health Care Equipment Suppliers

All these companies publish catalogs. Write for them; then compare prices and values.

Abbey Medical
(check phone book for nearest office)
800-421-5126; in California, 800-262-1294
One of the largest and most complete lines of home health care equipment available. Abbey, however, will only accept orders from health care professionals. You cannot order from them directly.

American Foundation for the Blind
Consumer Products Catalog
15 West 16th Street
New York, NY 10011
201-862-8838
Many useful supplies for the handicapped, especially for the visually handicapped.

Arthritis Self Help Products Catalog
Aids for Arthritis, Inc.
3 Little Knoll Court
Medford, NJ 08055
609-654-6918
Many excellent and ingenious around-the-house self-help aids for the physically disabled and handicapped.

Carolina Health and Fitness
Carolina Biological Supply Co.
2700 York Road
Burlington, NC 27215
919-584-0381
Health products with an emphasis on fitness but with some products for the bedridden and handicapped.

Cleo, Inc.
    3957 Mayfield Road
    Cleveland, OH 44121
    800-321-0595; local Ohio number: 216-382-7900
    Excellent selection of aids and self-help devices for the retail consumer.

HSA Health Supplies of America
    P.O. Box 288
    Farmville, NC 27828
    800-334-1187
    Perhaps the best of the consumer mail order medical supply catalogs. Wide range of orthopedic and exercise equipment, aids for grooming, skin care, first aid, and daily living.

Medical Self-Care Catalog
    1 Self-Care Center
    P.O. Box 130
    Mandeville, LA 70448
    504-892-8032
    Constantly expanding line of interesting and sometimes offbeat home care and self-care medical equipment.

Fred Sammons, Inc.
    P.O. Box 32
    Brookfield, IL 60513
    800-323-5547
    Along with Abbey, one of the largest and best stocked of the medical supply houses. Like Abbey, all equipment must be purchased through a health care professional. The company will not accept direct orders.

Sears Home Health Care
    (through your local Sears store)
    Good general line of home health care supplies. Most of their goods can be purchased directly from their stores. Catalogs issued.

Spenco Medical Corporation
    P.O. Box 2501
    Waco, TX 76702
    800-433-3334
    Sports medicine mostly, but with some useful home care equipment too.

4

Practical Home Care Concerns for Caregivers

You and your family are quite right. The home is the best place for your loved ones to get the kind of personalized, sensitive care that they deserve and that only you and your family can provide. The friendly pictures on the wall, the yummy smells coming from the kitchen, the familiar squeaks in the banister, all are immensely reassuring to ailing persons on many levels.

Although the intention is right, however, many caregivers are unprepared for the tasks that lie ahead. These tasks include both the emotional struggles that nursing demented persons inevitably brings, and the actual nursing skills and physical exertions that caregivers will eventually be expected to provide.

In the early days these demands are relatively manageable. Demented persons still have many coping skills in decent working order. They can look after their own bodies with relative efficiency, and they can make their needs known. Later on, in a year, in two years, in five years, in seven years, the going gets tougher. Then caregivers really need to know their turf. The early days are the time to find out about it and to prepare.

In Part III we delve into the psychological and emotional issues that crop up for caregivers during the duration of a typical senile dementia. Here, in the remainder of Part II, we deal with more tangible matters, with the hands-on stuff that patient care is made of—feeding, sleeping, exercise, bathing, grooming, dressing, and other nursing protocols—all of which are basic to effective home care.

Members of the staff at the Brookdale Center on Aging have spent a great deal of time at respite centers and in family residences, teaching caregivers ways of performing these tasks to maximum efficiency. The Brookdale people have come to realize that a family's job can be made remarkably easier if provided with the basics of home care information, plus a few simple nursing tricks and a working repertoire of clinical methods. Distilled from the experience gathered by Brookdale's teaching and respite staff over many years, what is presented here is the product of much trial, some error, and numberless hours spent with patients in various stages of dementia. Read it carefully, step by step. Though no single technique can move a mountain, these methods really do save time and relieve frustration when practiced collectively. As a teacher at one of the Brookdale home care seminars told her students, "Never underestimate the power of many small stratagems to reduce the weight of one huge burden."

Helping the Person Dress

Note the distinction between dressing a person and helping that person dress. This difference between *doing* and *helping* is a critical one and should be kept in mind throughout the duration of an individual's illness. Indeed, if a credo for AD caregivers could be written in stone, it would read something like this:

> I will do everything I can to make sure that whatever mental and physical capacities my loved one still possesses are used to their fullest, so that the maximum quality of life can be sustained at the highest possible plateau for the longest period of time.

Such an approach will give a sizable boost to the sick person's confidence and self-respect, and it will make your job considerably easier as well. Constant encouragement, reminding, and urging will be necessary to carry off this goal; so will the exertion of your will at times, to force demented persons to do things they would rather have you do for them. But the results will be well worth it for everyone. In short, you as caregiver are obliged to do everything in your power to help your loved ones help themselves.

One of the best times to encourage self-reliance is during the dressing ritual. If possible, let patients dress themselves every morning and undress themselves every night. This may sound like a formidable task for sick persons to accomplish, and often it is; but if you simplify both the procedure and the clothes themselves, as outlined here, self-dressing will become feasible for most patients, especially those in the earlier stages. Here is what to do:

1. Adapt clothes for easier putting on and wearing. Hard-to-manage zippers can be removed and replaced with Velcro tabs. Insert an elastic seam at the waist so that cumbersome belts are unnecessary. Buttons are a particular cause of frustration and are best replaced with Velcro tabs. Patients often have trouble keeping objects in their pockets; one deep pocket sewn onto all trousers, slacks, and dresses will help. Bear in mind too that some AD sufferers tend to put on considerable weight and others tend to lose it. Clothes should lend themselves to alterations in either direction.

2. Demented persons can be exceedingly rough on clothes, and any tight spots or pressure areas will quickly become vulnerable to rips and tears. Some persons take great delight in pulling at their clothes or ripping them apart. Strong, plain, baggy coverings are generally best.

3. Clothes should be easy to slip in and out of and should be selected according to a person's specific needs. For women who are physically handicapped, pajamas are especially difficult to wear; use a nightgown instead, one that slips over the shoulders and head. Don't expect persons to figure out how to put on button shirts. Supply pullover sweaters, polo shirts, or sweatshirts instead. Special easy-snap-on shoes can be purchased from some shoe stores or from orthopedic supply houses.

4. Being neatly dressed will help a sick person's self-esteem. Conversely, sloppy dress with trousers at half-mast or a sweater that flops open at the breasts will be demeaning for you, if not for the patient. To the best of your ability, keep the person's wardrobe updated and their clothes tidy, color-coordinated, and free of embarrassing stains. Though it may sound obvious, make sure pants and shirts are not worn inside out or backward and that all socks match—it won't be obvious to an AD sufferer. Hear one caregiver on this subject:

When Carl was healthy, he was a sharp dresser, and though he has Alzheimer's disease now, I find that he seems still to like the feel of nice clean clothes on his body. He enjoys running his hands over linen pants and gets a happy look on his face when he rubs the fabric in a cotton sweater. I know that somewhere in his mind he's pleased when I make a fuss over how he looks, though he doesn't say anything. In his well days he would never think of going out without a coat and tie. So I make sure he has one on whenever we visit his sister or go out for dinner at a restaurant. He can't tie a tie much now, of course, so I put one of those cute clip-on numbers on him. When his hair is combed and he's all dressed up, he still cuts a handsome figure.

5. Though patients should be encouraged to dress themselves, you will want to prevent them from potential hazards such as falls or sudden disorientation. Pay special attention whenever a person's balance or orientation becomes imperiled, as when stepping into or out of trousers, pulling a shirt or sweater over the head, or bending down to put on shoes. Some home care aides insist that their patients be seated whenever they dress. Others stand next to them during the dressing process to provide support. It is also a good idea to have the person dress in the same part of the room every day and to have this area well padded with a rug on the floor, all sharp edges and corners protected, at least one object available to grab onto for steadiness if necessary, and enough light to see what is going on.

6. Clothes in the sick person's closet and bureau drawers should be arranged so that they are easy to take out and put back. Make sure no awkward stretching is required; reaching can cause persons to lose their balance. Too many clothes crammed into a small space is a bewildering sight for AD sufferers and may trigger a frustration response. Try laying out the day's clothes on the bed ahead of time each morning. While persons are putting on their clothes, hand them each article of clothing as it is needed. This will make dressing easier and will shield the persons from the potential discombobulations that forced decisions bring. Edna has taken care of her sister Nancy for eleven months:

> *Edna:* My sister Nancy had three dresses dangling in her closet last week. She wasn't sure which one to choose. She agonized over the choice for what seemed like an hour, then went ahead and put on all three dresses, one over the other. The next day I took all her stuff out of the closet and left only the dress that I decided she should wear that Monday. Now she's got no choice but to put on the right dress. This simplified the matter to the point where she could deal with the dressing challenge in an easy way. If you want one piece of advice about dressing, it would be this: Don't put them in the position of having to make a choice. You do it for them.

7. When arranging a person's clothes, sort them by type: All socks in one drawer, all shirts in another, all underpants in a third. Compartmentalizing makes it easier for both you and the demented person. Just be sure not to switch the designated areas around once they are estab-

lished: The sock drawer is *always* for socks, the slip drawer *always* for slips, and so on.

8. To help maintain a sense of self-determination while dressing, consult with persons beforehand concerning the style and type of clothing they prefer. Questions like "Do you want to wear red or blue?" or "Which do you like today, Mom, the skirt or slacks?" can supply AD sufferers with a much-needed sense of participation and control. Persons who were fashion-conscious before their sickness will enjoy being consulted on these issues now; they will surprise you at times with sudden flashes of taste and discrimination.

9. One trick for eliminating awkward dressing combinations is to make sure that all items of clothing in the closet and the drawers are design-coordinated. For example, if one item has stripes on it, be sure that nothing else in the same storage area will clash with it. If one blouse is green, be sure all available slacks are of a complementary color. If possible, limit the wardrobe to just three or four compatible colors: a few cheerful greens, yellows, and browns will do. This guarantees that all clothes are stylistically interchangeable and that whatever combinations the person happens to choose will automatically look right.

10. The person will put on whatever clothes you put on display, so arrange the wardrobe according to the season. Have only summer clothes available during summer, winter clothes during winter. Keep the scarves and boots well out of sight in the warm months, the Bermuda shorts and T-shirts locked away when it is snowing.

11. Conduct a thorough dress check before taking the person out in public. One respite site coordinator at Brookdale reported that several of her patients showed up consistently wearing bedroom slippers or missing their socks. Another talked about trousers being worn inside out. These embarrassing gaffs could have been prevented before leaving the house by sharp-eyed caregivers.

12. Wash-and-wear clothes will eliminate the need for ironing. Sneakers, easy to clean in the washing machine, are especially suitable if the person is both ambulatory and incontinent. Machine-washable garments are preferable to those that require dry cleaning. Spots, stripes, and simple patterns hide stains and reduce the need for constant laundering. Reversible clothes will help prevent embarrassment should the person put clothes on inside out.

13. Demented persons sometimes fixate on a particular shirt or pair of pants. Suddenly they *must* wear this article of clothing every day; nothing else will do. They will tell you that all other clothes in their

closet "don't belong to me! They belong to someone else! Throw them away!" If the person can still read, name tapes sewn into all clothing may help convince them that the clothes really are their own. If you absolutely cannot dissuade the person from wearing the same shirt and pants every day, purchase duplicates and switch them whenever it is time to launder or replace the originals.

14. Mechanical dressing aids for the handicapped are available from several mail order medical suppliers. Though in many cases these gadgets will be too complicated for AD persons to maneuver, such items as long-handled shoehorns for putting on shoes without bending down, a zipper pull for easier grasp on the zipper, and one-handed shoelace fasteners may be of value to persons in the early stages, and then later on to caregivers when helping persons dress. These and other aids for dressing are available from the Cleo, Inc., catalog (3957 Mayfield Road, Cleveland, OH 44121; 800-321-0595).

Nutrition and Menu

It is impossible to say in advance whether a demented person's appetite will increase or decrease. Even at the advanced stages of AD, desire for food can be formidable, and occasionally it runs totally out of control. In such cases the neurological mechanism that controls the appestat becomes dysfunctional, causing the person to gorge without cease, stopping only when all eatables are removed from sight.

At the opposite extreme, some persons will become maddeningly picky eaters, focusing on three or four particular foods and refusing to accept anything else. Whatever the situation, some conflict is likely to arise over food. Here are some helpful tips:

• You may discover that patients shun their food not because of insufficient appetite but because the knives and forks are too difficult to manipulate. To compensate for loss of digital dexterity, serve finger foods as frequently as possible—sandwiches, hamburgers, carrot or celery sticks, fish sticks, french fries, cucumber bits, chicken legs, ice cream sandwiches, bread and butter, corn on the cob, diced apples, bananas, orange and pineapple slices, pizza, and hot dogs. If the sick person is still able to use utensils, spoons are easier to manipulate than forks and are less dangerous.

• Instead of having three large meals every day, during which the person's attention wanders and interest in food lags, serving a number of small meals throughout the day may help get more food down.

• Demented persons often feel infantilized when caretakers cut their food for them at the table. If this occurs, do all the preparation in the kitchen, then present the food after it has been sliced.

• Tailor your eating plans to the person's specific habits. If the sick person's appetite is uncontrolled, serve discrete portions and remove all extra food from sight. If the person tends to play with food, make it difficult to get at by serving it in a bowl with a half-closed lid. Some persons are hoarders and must be carefully watched while they eat; they may hide food under the table or try to smuggle it back to their rooms. People who enjoyed particular foods before they were ill tend to retain those preferences. Thus one of the best ways to get demented patients to eat is to do what you did before: Serve them what they like.

• Sloppy spills will be frequent at the table, and you must be prepared to accept the fact that demented persons will not sup according to Emily Post. Always keep a few napkins handy for cleaning hands and mouths (in the later stages, persons may even smear food on their cheeks or rub it on their heads). A mat placed beneath the place where the person eats will catch all fallen residues. An easy-to-clean plastic table-cloth is also useful. Straws will make drinking neater for you and easier for the person. Spills can be controlled by using untippable or "snorkel" cups, high-rimmed plates, suction cups to keep dinnerware fastened to the table, and large bibs. Check the HSA and Cleo, Inc., catalogs for these and other eating aids such as weighted spoons, one-hand cutlery, drinking glass holders, double-handed drinking cups, scooper dishes, and terry cloth bibs. Cleo, Inc., also sells a 267-page book called *Mealtime Manual for the Aged and Handicapped* that describes how kitchen and eating tasks can be specially adapted to the needs of the handicapped aged. (Catalog information appears at the end of Chapter 3.)

• In the later stages, persons may tend to eat without chewing their food adequately. You may literally have to remind them to chew after every bite, and even then the hazard potential is high. The best way around this dilemma is to cut food into small pieces or, better yet, serve soft or semiliquid foods that can be eaten with a minimum of mastication. After consulting with your physician concerning diet, think along the lines of preparing such foods as soups, whipped potatoes, juices, meats put through a meat grinder, puddings, soufflés, creamed or puréed vegetables, and applesauce. Hand-operated food grinders are excellent for pulping fruits and vegetables.

• Demented persons tend to be extremely imitative. When you

stand, they stand; when you sit, they sit. And what you eat, they will eat too. This imitation reflex can be used to your advantage at the table where the sight of several family members enthusiastically digging into meals will trigger the AD person to follow suit. If the person is sitting and dawdling, get the person's attention, pick up your spoon, scoop up a piece of food, and put it in your mouth, looking the person directly in the eye. Then tell the person to do the same. This trick often produces instant results.

● Persons who are still functional should not be allowed to eat by themselves. Studies have shown that patients who eat alone or who are segregated from the family table at mealtime tend to be more erratic in their eating habits and less well nourished. Eating with loved ones can provide a pleasant and much-needed emotional perk.

● If the person is a skimpy eater and you want to increase his or her daily nutritional intake, you can "sneak" extra nutrients into the diet. When you cook hamburgers, add wheat germ to the mixture. Several fresh eggs can be put into a chocolate soda or a soup. Chopped celery and carrots mix nicely with tuna salad. A little lemon juice adds extra vitamin C to lettuce. Grind up sunflower seeds or almonds and sprinkle them over breakfast cereal. Health care workers report that demented patients tend to enjoy foods that contain bananas or snacks that are banana-flavored. Keep bowls of fruit on display, or platters of sliced vegetables and mixed nuts. Demented persons especially enjoy sweet foods, fruits, and ice cream (you can make the ice cream more nutritional by sprinkling it with fruit and almonds).

● Eventually it may become necessary to hand-feed a bedbound person at every meal. When this moment arrives, the following steps will make the process easier:

1. Prop the person up with pillows into a comfortable sitting position. Never feed persons while they are lying down; they may choke. If propping up a person's entire body is impractical, at least elevate the head.

2. Cover the person's pillow and bedding with a protective washable covering.

3. Make sure hot foods are not too hot, cold foods not too cold. Be especially careful of hot liquids. Test a few drops on your wrist before feeding.

4. The foods you serve should be well pulped and should demand

a minimum of chewing. They can be puréed and, if necessary, strained. Sometimes completely liquefied foods will be best. Consult with your doctor for instructions.

5. Fill the spoon about two-thirds full, bring it up to the person's mouth, apply slight pressure on the bottom lip so that the person will open voluntarily, then tip the food in. Allow at least five seconds for the person to swallow.

6. Serve all liquids via a straw or drinking tube. Place the straw in the person's mouth, keeping the sipping end above the level of the liquid so that air bubbles are avoided. Support the person's head while drinking.

7. Talk quietly to the person during feeding. Give encouragement. Don't hurry the process.

8. Whatever small things persons can do for themselves at this stage should be encouraged. Sometimes they will be able to hold a cup or guide a spoon to their mouth. Root them on.

9. Maintain an eating chart. Record the times of day the person has eaten, the amount of food taken in, and any notable reactions. Make a record of any foods that are especially liked or disliked. Jot down the times of day when the person's appetite is strong or weak.

Toilet

In the early to middle stages of Alzheimer's disease and other chronic dementias, most sufferers are still able to use the toilet facilities on their own, though often with some gentle and forbearing help from the caregiver. Sometimes the person simply forgets where the bathroom is located. A large picture of a toilet on the bathroom door will help in this regard, as will strips of reflecting tape and a night light. Sometimes caregivers will have to accompany persons into the bathroom, helping them to remove underclothes and to get comfortably seated. Each person's needs will be different.

Embarrassment concerning toilet activities dies hard, sometimes last in a person's social consciousness. It is not unusual for persons who have lost all semblance of shame when it comes to exposing their privates or to causing a scene in a public place to remain quite diffident concerning their need for privacy in the bathroom. Robby B., a young man serving as a volunteer at an Alzheimer's respite facility, spent a good part of his workday standing by the door of the men's bathroom helping persons when help was needed. One morning a man whose symptoms were moderately advanced and who was given to sudden outbursts of temper entered the bathroom and remained inside for an inordinately long period of time. Finally Robby went in to investigate. There he found the man, pants down, tears in his eyes, face flushed with anger and mortification. In front of him was a toilet, a large white trash bin, and a sink. All three were white receptacles; the man could not tell them apart.

Sensing the delicacy of the situation and wishing to help the man save face, Robby cleared his throat, touched the man on the shoulder, and quietly said, "Sorry to interrupt you, Mr. N., but I see that you haven't finished yet. I've made the same mistake myself." He then gently pushed the man in the direction of the toilet, announcing, "I see you're about to go to the bathroom in this toilet (touches the toilet). I guess you'll want to put the seat down when you do (raises and lowers the toilet seat), and then you'll want to pull up your pants when you're finished (mimics pulling up his pants). You can wash your hands in that sink afterwards if you like (walks over to the sink and turns on the tap)."

Notice that Robby assiduously avoided using the word *help* when addressing the man and that he made every effort to make the man feel that he was actually doing it all by himself.

Toilet care, in other words, is a potentially awkward issue that touches on primal distastes and anxious privacies on both sides of the patient-caregiver axis. Caregivers will no doubt be obliged to perform many off-putting jobs such as removing soiled underpants or helping patients wipe themselves; patients may themselves feel exposed and infantilized at these moments. Clearly, this task must be approached with forbearance, tact, and, above all, knowledge of the specific methods that will minimize embarrassment and maximize efficiency. From the caregiver's perspective, the goals should be to keep their loved ones continent as long as possible and at the same time to make sure that their bathroom experience is safe, comfortable, and hygienic. The following methods will help:

• Keep a written list of the hours at which patients are accustomed to using the bathroom. At what times of day do they urinate? How many hours separate urinations? How many times a day, or a week, do they eliminate? Look for patterns. Note all exceptions. Keep track of all times.

• Next, encourage persons to defecate and urinate *only* at these accustomed times. Discourage toilet activity at odd or random hours. Once every one to three days is average for bowel movements, every two or three hours for urination. Reminders can be provided after every meal, on rising in the morning, and on going to bed at night.

Keeping the person to an exact routine may prove difficult at first; later, when persons no longer associate the pressure to evacuate with the actual need to use the toilet, it becomes impossible. In many instances, however, over the days and weeks, bowels and bladders may accommodate themselves to the fixed schedule you impose, and eventually the regime should become second nature. Toilet activity then becomes more predictable, and the chances of accidental self-soiling are accordingly reduced. Note that peristaltic activity is strongest in the morning; encourage bowel movements at this time to reduce the chance of incontinent slips later in the day.

• Demented persons who can no longer talk may still try to indicate bathroom urges via behavioral clues. It's then up to you to decipher the code. Some will hitch at their pants or make funny rocking motions. Others will point to their rear ends or make the sound of breaking wind. Many persons become agitated and restless when nature calls, and when they do, if the agitation coincides with the person's usual toilet times, assume that toileting is the issue.

• When the person enters the bathroom, provide visual and auditory cues as reminders of the purpose of the visit. Flush the toilet several times. Point out where the toilet paper is located. Turn the water on in the sink. Lower the toilet seat. Explain why the person is in the bathroom and what must be done there. You may have to talk the person through the process, although sometimes just helping raise a dress or lower pants will be enough of a cue and the person will take it from there.

• Regulate the person's diet in such a way that it keeps toilet habits regular and predictable. For instance, serving meals at the same time each day will produce bowel movements at predictable intervals. Do not give too many liquids at night; too much to drink will invite bed wetting. Learn how long it takes laxative foods such as prunes or sauerkraut to take effect; then plan accordingly.

• Alzheimer's persons sometimes have trouble finding the bathroom or telling a toilet bowl from other round, empty bathroom objects. Christina's husband was appalled when Christina started moving her bowels one day into the large clay living room flowerpot where the ficus tree was planted. Somehow the associations of the pot's roundness and the dirt in the bowl triggered the message "defecate," and Christina obeyed. Like so many other demented persons at this stage of illness, Christina dimly recalled the procedure but forgot the details; she remembered that people are supposed to relieve themselves into an oval receptacle. She simply lost track of what kind.

Marking bathrooms with signs and pictures or painting the bathroom door with bright colors will help in cases of mistaken identity, as will careful supervision, especially during the hours of the day when the person is accustomed to toileting. When the time arrives, ask persons if they have to go, lead them to the bathroom, help them with whatever dressing or undressing is required, then wait outside until the process is finished, or until the person needs your help.

• Bathroom problems tend to arise only for a limited number of reasons. Just as parents determine why an infant is crying by ticking off a few standard possibilities—illness, pain, needs sleep, needs changing—so can you often get to the bottom of a toilet dilemma by asking yourself the following questions:

1. Does the person know where the bathroom is located?
2. Does the person still know how to use the toilet, or does he or she need reminding?
3. Does the person have enough stamina to reach the bathroom from where he or she usually sits?
4. Can the person exercise self-control from the time the urge occurs to the time he or she reaches the toilet?
5. Can the person still identify the physical urge to eliminate, and can he or she connect it to the need to go to the bathroom?
6. Is the person hardy enough to sit up on the toilet without support? Is falling a potential problem?
7. Is the person constipated? Sick? Is there indication of bowel trouble of some kind?

Constipation

Constipation occurs frequently among people who are inactive, heavily medicated, or confined to bed. There are several lines of defense against it:

• Include plenty of fiber in the person's meals, plenty of fresh fruits and vegetables, grains, and bran cereal. Foods high in natural fiber include apples, avocados, beets, corn, green beans, grits, lentils, mangoes, parsnips, potatoes in their skins, raspberries, rolled oats, and strawberries.

• If tolerated, foods that ferment quickly in the stomach are excellent natural laxatives. These include sauerkraut, cabbage juice, and sourdough bread. For some people a mixture of half sauerkraut juice and half tomato juice, with a squeeze of lemon added, will do the trick.

● Eliminate foods that cause constipation, such as chocolate, refined sugars, and fatty meats. Substitute unrefined, unprocessed grains for the refined varieties: brown rice for white, whole wheat bread for white bread. Use natural laxative foods such as yogurt, stewed fruit, cabbage and leafy greens, pumpkin seeds, papaya juice, prunes and prune juice, rhubarb, apricots, ground flaxseed, and bran products.

● Make sure the person drinks several glasses of water a day. Nothing constipates faster than dehydration. A glass of warm water a few minutes after waking up will encourage a strong morning evacuation. Exercise will help too, stimulating the alimentary tract and invigorating the organs of elimination. (Effective exercise plans for AD persons are provided in Chapter 6.) For some persons, massaging the abdomen in slow, deep, circular clockwise motions also helps.

● If natural aids don't do the trick, consult with your physician about laxatives. If the doctor approves, start with the natural variety. So-called bulk-forming laxatives are made mostly from organic substances and work surprisingly well in cases of mild constipation. Wheat bran and oat bran, two of the best, can be added to cereals or meat preparations. Buy them at natural food stores. Psyllium derivatives like Metamucil, Siblin, and Mucilose are available at most drugstores, along with a useful malt soup extract known as Maltsupex. Have the patient take these preparations with plenty of water. If you intend to mix them with aspirin or prescription drugs, consult with your physician first.

● If bulk-forming laxatives don't do the trick, stool softeners such as Bu-Lax, D-S-S, and Colace will help, but give them only for one or two days in a row at most. Lubricant laxatives such as mineral oil are sometimes appropriate, though overuse will interfere with proper nutrient absorption (and be careful—mineral oil taken at bedtime can occasionally run back up the esophagus and be drawn into the lungs). Suppositories work for many constipation sufferers, but demented persons will often be ornery about using them. Saline laxatives such as milk of magnesia and tartar salts trigger the loss of important body salts among the elderly and are not frequently recommended.

● The most powerful laxatives of all are the so-called stimulant laxatives. These act directly on the intestines, speeding up peristalsis and artificially reducing the time food takes to move through the bowels. Castor oil, bile salts, phenolphthalein (Ex-Lax, Feen-a-Mint, Phenolox), senna (Senexon, Senokot), and bisacodyl (Cenalax, Fleet Bisacodyl,

Bisco-Lax) are all in this category. Ordinarily, it is recommended that persons be given stimulant laxatives only on rare occasions, and then only if they are absolutely needed, as in cases of impaction. Never use these powerful drugs for more than three or four days at a time. They work too well—the AD person's bowels will quickly become dependent on them.

Bedpans, Urinals, and Commodes

If persons are partially incontinent or bedbound and incapable of regular trips to the bathroom, bedpans and urinals are required. Keep these items near the incontinent person at all times but out of sight and well covered. When they are needed, help the person sit up, prop him or her up with supports, and place the pan under the person's hips. The whole technique takes a bit of doing and varies with sex, age, weight, and physical condition. Before you attempt it on your own, it is wise to take a lesson or two from an experienced caregiver or a health care pro. Have toilet paper handy, and remove the pan promptly after use. Empty the contents into the toilet, and cleanse the receptacle thoroughly with soap and hot water.

Commodes or portable toilets are sometimes appropriate, usually when the person is traveling or out of bed but cannot easily get to a bathroom. If using a commode, keep it within fetching distance and avoid placing it in unusual spots around the house. Turning a section of the living room into a toilet area may be handy as far as proximity goes, but in the sick person's mind this abrupt change of location can be disorienting. Commode chairs may be purchased or rented from medical supply houses. Some Red Cross chapters maintain a loan service through which commode chairs can be borrowed for extended periods of time.

Incontinence

The time may come when the person will no longer associate the physical impulse to eliminate with the act of going to the toilet. If and when this occurs—it doesn't always—soiling of the clothes will be a natural consequence, and steps must be taken.

Bear in mind, however, that incontinence, both the bladder and bowel varieties, can sometimes be a temporary condition, resulting from medication, a urinary tract infection, diabetes, a stomach ailment, even a stroke. It is not necessarily caused by brain degeneration per se and may thus not necessarily be permanent. Consult with your physician on this matter before taking steps to counter the incontinence. If the condition is temporary or occasional, your doctor may not want the patient to use protective pads for fear of making the person reliant on them.

Urinary Incontinence. As a rule, urinary incontinence begins before bowel incontinence and is a good deal easier to control. Absorbent pads worn during the times of day when wetting most often takes place will keep the person comfortable and dry. Before assuming that a loved one is helplessly wetting his or her pants, however, caregivers should be certain that the person is not simply "dribbling," a common condition among the elderly, both sick and well. Dribbling can take place when exercising, coughing, standing up, or moving around at a quick pace. If a correlation can be made between these daily actions and wetting, the problem may then be viewed as the consequences of age and not as incontinence per se.

Find out also if wetting stems from actual lack of bladder control or if it is due to the fact that no one happens to be around to bring the person to the toilet when nature calls. Limiting a person's daily fluid intake will help in this regard, especially at night, when wetting most frequently occurs. Note too that some reports claim that a bit of bold-faced bribery will also help keep wetting under control. Nurses have found, for example, that by offering patients pieces of candy in return for waiting a certain amount of time between urinations, incontinence can be stemmed. This technique is not in the nursing books, but if it works, go for it!

Bed Wetting. Though occasional bed wetting occurs even in the early stages of dementia, it may become increasingly frequent as the dementia progresses. When and if the person is bedridden, the bladder and lower extremity muscles will become correspondingly weakened. This coupled with a lessened ability to recognize the toilet urge will soon make nighttime incontinence a rule rather than an exception. Besides restricting fluid intake at night and establishing a regular every-two-or-three-hour toileting program as described, protective bedding, rubber or plastic sheets, and, if the person is still able to use it, a commode by the bed will all help.

Bowel Incontinence. Bowel incontinence is, of course, more serious than urinary incontinence and when it starts it is often irreversible. However, though accidents may happen even during the mild stages of dementia (note that fecal impaction can sometimes explain bowel incontinence in the early stages), regular daily soilings usually occur only when the person has lost all physiological sense of cause and effect. Incontinence pads and protective bedding will be necessary at this stage (not "diapers," as some caregivers refer to them—sometimes, insensitively, in front of the patient), and it will be smart on the caregiver's part to receive instruction from a professional on how to put these coverings on and take them off. Helpful also are incontinence pants, washable polyester or vinyl-coated nylon knits that contain a stay-dry lining and a leakproof pouch that holds absorbent disposable pads. Adult protective pads and pants are available at drugstores and medical supply houses.

Finally, cleanliness and hygiene are of utmost importance in cases of incontinence. After using the pads, dispose of them, wipe the soiled area clean, wash it thoroughly, and towel it dry gently. Note that urine deposits leave traces of ammonia on sensitive skin areas, and these can lead to bedsores and infections. Wash all groin areas carefully, and apply a soothing ointment before fastening on a fresh pad. The aim here is to ensure dryness, prevent spotting on clothes, and keep the person's body free from dirt, infection, and disagreeable odors. Daily baths will be mandatory to accomplish this goal (see the next section), as will regular changes of clothes.

Bathroom Equipment for the Disabled

Toilet aids for the handicapped are available from most major health equipment supply houses. Practically mandatory for many demented persons are raised toilet seats and toilet seats with safety rails. These come in all sizes and can be ordered directly by mail, sometimes through a hospital or an orthopedic supply store. Also available are reusable incontinence pants (Cleo, Inc.), male and female urinals (Cleo, Inc.), folding commodes, carrying cases for elevated toilet seats (Cleo, Inc.), and commode wheelchairs (Abbey). Addresses of the supply houses are given at the end of Chapter 3.

Bathing

The bathroom safety devices described in Chapter 3—grab bars, mats, nonskid tape—will all be needed if your loved one is to be bathed regularly at home. Just remember that you will have to remind demented persons each time to use these aids, to reach for the grab bar in the tub or to step on the rubber mat; they will not remember on their own. In general, persons in the early stages of dementia will usually be able to bathe themselves, perhaps with a little help from their friends.

Let bathing become an automatic part of the person's routine and schedule it, ideally, for the same hour each day. Even persons who are resistant to bathing will get used to this regular event if it is built into their routine, and after a while they will acquiesce. Bathroom aids will help in this campaign and can be ordered from medical supply houses or orthopedic pharmacies. Helpful items for demented persons include long-handled sponges, curved bath brushes, hand sponges, sponge or loofah wash mitts, back scrubbers, tub safety benches and rails, portable hand showers, safety mats, self-adhering treads, and wall grab bars. If ordering by mail, Cleo, Abbey, HSA, Sammons, Carolina, and Sears each carry a full line of home care bathing equipment. Ordering information is supplied at the end of Chapter 3.

Sometimes, of course, it is just plain impossible to talk persons into taking a bath or shower, and many caregivers report hair-pulling frustrations in this area. In response to what appears to be an almost universal dilemma, the staff members of the Source for Nursing Home Literature in Columbus, Ohio, have put forth several interesting suggestions in their recent literature. Their advice is well taken and well worth passing along. In summary, caretakers are advised as follows:*

1. Allow demented persons a degree of choice in the bathing process. Don't simply say, "Take a bath." Say, "It's time to bathe. Do you want to take a bath or a shower?"

2. Persons often rebel against bathing not because they don't enjoy the experience but because they are angered by the fact that they can't remember how it is done. Caregivers can alleviate this frustration by presenting the bathing process to patients one step at a time. For instance, start by filling the tub. Then bring in the robe and slippers. Then help the person get undressed. Then help him or her into the water. Then hand over the soap, then the washcloth and sponge, and so forth. While you're doing it, describe each step out loud and identify every action: "Now I'm turning on the water. Now I'm going to give you the soap. . . ." In this way you break the process down into manageable

* Dorothy Coons, Lena Metzelaar, Anne Robinson, Beth Spencer, eds., *A Better Life* (Columbus, Ohio: Source for Nursing Home Literature, 1986).

increments, and for the patient the experience becomes accordingly controllable and comprehensible.

3. Post a chart on the bathroom door that records the times and dates of each bath. This way when tub time arrives, the person cannot object that "I just took a bath!"

4. Promise a reward. Assure persons that if they take a bath now, they will be given a piece of candy later on, a walk outside, or some other pleasure.

Giving a Bath

In general, baths are considered safer than showers. Caregivers have a good deal more control if patients are sitting upright in a tub, and patients are less likely to slip in this position. Several Brookdale-trained professionals have remarked that demented persons tend to be frightened by showers and that they perceive the violent, down-coming streams of water as a threatening bombardment. For those who are addicted to showers and who resist the notion of taking a bath, a hose shower attachment that fits over the faucet and allows persons to take a shower while sitting in the tub may be the best compromise. Whatever you do, however, opt if possible for baths. This is important.

Run the tub water, test its temperature, then fill the tub no more than one-third full. If your loved one is able to undress, have him or her do so (if shy about being naked in front of you, the person may wear shorts or underpants). Provide body support if needed, and help the person step into the tub while keeping a firm grip on the grab bar.

Hold the person by the waist as he or she slides into the water. This is another nursing maneuver that is best learned from a health care professional. You will definitely want to make practice runs with a healthy volunteer before trying it on the patient. But however you do it, be careful: When walking on slippery tiles and smooth porcelain, even the most alert elderly person is vulnerable to falls.

Never leave a demented patient alone in the tub. You or other family members should stay in close proximity. Make sure the person does not aspirate water and, if needed, help the person wash. Hot baths can be enormously calming for demented persons and can provide caregivers with a longed-for respite. Lee S. told us that whenever he gives his wife a bath, he brings a chair and a favorite magazine into the bathroom and catches up on his reading while his wife plays in the water, sometimes for hours.

Should demented persons be given toys while bathing? Some experts say yes, some no. Toys will infantilize but also entertain. Lee S. told us, "If I can keep my wife in a tub for forty-five minutes with cups and a boat that floats, I do it. She likes it and I like it." There are really no rules on this one. Do as you see fit.

Sometimes the person must be bathed in bed. In this instance, caretakers should be even more regular with their washings than before, as bedridden persons desperately require the therapeutic and hygienic assets that a bath can bring. Besides cleaning the whole body and reducing potentially dangerous bacteria, bed baths relax and revive patients, raise their spirits, and provide them with a limited amount of exercise.

To give a bed bath, first, make sure that the person's bedroom is warm and that protective rubber or plastic coverings are laid over the sheets and pillow. Fill a large basin with warm water. Have soap handy, a washcloth, several towels, toilet articles as needed, and a change of nightclothes. Wet the washcloth, wring it out, make a kind of bath mitt by folding it into a square, add a little soap to the mitt, and wash the person's body entirely, starting with the ears and proceeding to the face, chin, arms, hands, chest, abdomen, hips, groin, legs, and feet. After washing each area, rinse the washcloth and go over the area a second time to remove excess soap. Wash with long, firm strokes, and bear down firmly on body parts that need special cleaning—between the toes, under the armpits, behind the ears, and in the groin.

When the bath is finished, help the person change into a fresh set of nightclothes. Remove wet linens and protective coverings from the bed, and cover the person up. You might now consider giving the person a massage with fragrant oils or talcum powder, a taxing job, perhaps, but one of the best of all ways to communicate with—and comfort—a bedbound person.

Massage

Massage is perhaps the most intimate resource in the caregiver's tool chest. Long after demented persons' minds have given up, their bodies remain amazingly receptive to the reassuring signals communicated through the touch of a loving caregiver.

Massage for a demented person is not your usual clubhouse massage. *Gently*, *firmly*, and *slowly* are the orders of the day; a too enthusiastic rub may be translated as a physical assault. Start on the back using deep circular and stroking motions; then proceed to the arms and hands using long, firm strokes. End at the torso, legs, and feet. While massaging, use warm oil (being careful to put a protective sheet under the person to catch all drippings) or fresh-scented talcum powder. If a person's skin is especially dry, you can use a moisturizing emollient, providing skin care as well as relaxation. Long, firm strokes are best; forget about percussion or pounding, as such motions may frighten the subject. Remember too that the person's attention span will be limited, which means you should plan on massage sessions that last no longer than five or ten minutes.

Grooming

Another important way to keep everyone's spirits raised is by daily grooming. True it is, perhaps, that at a certain point in the disease process demented persons will lose interest in their appearance. But keep in mind the fact that you as caregiver must look at this person too. The truth of the matter is that if a loved one's hair is combed, face is washed, skin is moist, fingernails are cleaned, mouth is wiped, and body is kept free of odor, these cosmetic improvements will cause you as caregiver to look more favorably on your task. The reality of the situation is that no matter how much we love the sick person, we can still be turned off by their bad smells, dirty hair, disheveled clothes, scab-covered hands, open bedsores, and general slovenly look. It just works this way. Jeannette Richardson, a registered nurse and senior training associate at Brookdale, speaks on the subject:

Jeannette: Whenever I go into the home of a person with Alzheimer's disease, I tell the families that whatever the person used to do to take care of her body and appearance, she should keep on doing it. We want the person to look as normal as possible. If the person wore rouge and lipstick, keep it up. Don't stop now when she *really* needs it. Or, for instance, maybe I'd like my dad to come as close as possible to looking the way he did when he was well. So I tell the family: Keep him shaved. Clean him. Let him get dressed up now and then with a shirt and tie and nice jacket. If it's a woman, have her hair fixed. She can wear perfume or something nice to put on. If she comes to dinner in a freshly pressed skirt and blouse rather than a housedress, everyone at the table will find it more pleasant to have her there. You see, by having persons look presentable, the family will want to keep them at home longer. They won't be so [eager] to send them away to an institution.

When grooming an AD person, follow what home aides come to know during their training sessions as the three S's: *structure, supervise, simplify*. This trio of imperatives has application to practically every aspect of caregiving, especially to matters of personal hygiene and daily grooming.

Structure.   Provide grooming on a regular basis. Don't miss a day. Insist on it even if the person resists. Hair combed in the morning, afternoon, and night. Hair washed twice a week. Beard shaved every two days. Like clockwork. Skin anointed with cream once a day—dry skin itches, and scratching produces unsightly sores. Hands washed after every meal. Nails trimmed twice a month, hair cut periodically. Feet washed frequently and covered with talcum powder. Clothes changed on a regular basis. Deodorant applied every morning after washing. Establish a personal care regimen and do not deviate. It will keep the person alert longer and intact longer.

Supervise.   If persons can do things for themselves, let them; at the same time, supervise, but in a subtle way. When Margaret applies rouge to her lips, her aim is uneven at best, and sometimes odd streaks show up on her nose and chin. Still, her family encourages her to apply this makeup and only later, when she has forgotten how the lines got there, will they wipe them off. Help AD persons help themselves. Peter S. can now barely hold a comb. Yet he gets pleasure from having his hair combed and enjoys the sensation of running his fingers through his beautiful crop of white hair. His private nurse helps him do the job by taking his hand and helping him comb through his hair several times. Then she brings him a mirror, shows Peter his reflection, and compliments him on how nice he looks.

Simplify.   Make grooming jobs as easy to manage as possible. For instance, keep a person's hair short so that the hair-cutting procedure is simplified. Electric shavers are easier and safer to use than razors. Keep fingernails trimmed close to the quick so that manicures are unnecessary. Complicated caretaking jobs can be simplified by using mechanical home aids such as home hair-cutting kits (Sammons catalog), nostril and eyebrow clippers (Sammons), nail care combination sets (HSA catalog), and easy-grip hairbrushes (HSA). (Addresses of suppliers appear at the end of Chapter 3.)

Some Important Grooming Concerns

Skin Care.   Good nutrition is important for skin welfare, as is exercise and general body movement. Keep a person's skin well lubricated with moisturizers and emollients. Massage will improve skin tone and promote increased circulation, an especially important concern for invalids. If the person is bedridden, make sure there are no unnecessary ridges or lumps in the mattress and that the sheets are kept free from particles that can irritate the skin. The groin and armpits and, for large-breasted women, the cleft between the breasts tend to host bacteria. These areas must be kept especially clean and dry.

Pressure Sores.   Not exactly a grooming consideration, but certainly an issue of major concern for both appearance and health are the *decubiti,* pressure sores or bedsores that plague bedridden persons and at times become so severe that bone can be seen through the broken skin.

Bedsores develop from the pressure which is exerted on body parts by a mattress or a chair surface. This pressure reduces the circulation to the affected part and eventually causes its surface cells to die and erode. Like water wearing down stone, skin areas are slowly rubbed away until an opening or break occurs. For bedbound or chairbound persons who spend most of their time in a sitting position, the areas of greatest vulnerability include the heels and ankles, the back of the knees, the back of the thighs, the lower and middle back, and the elbows. Bedridden persons confined to the supine position develop decubiti on the heels, calves, buttocks, elbows, scapulae, and back of the head.

Once a skin ulcer has appeared, treatment can be difficult, and chances are a physician's help will be required. Better to avoid the problem early on by taking the proper preventive measures, which include these:

- A patient's position must be shifted approximately every two hours. Turn from the right side to the left or from a stomach position to a back position. Encourage persons to move as much and as often as possible on their own.
- Bacteria in fecal wastes makes skin highly susceptible to breakdown, and toxins quickly contribute to tissue erosion. The acids in urine are likewise lethal to skin surfaces and must be immediately washed away following every incontinent slip. Next to changes in body position, dryness is the most important preventive against

bedsores. All potential pressure sore areas of the body should be kept clean and well toweled.

- Periodically examine potential trouble areas on the sick person's body. Check the parts mentioned earlier with special attention, the buttocks, heels, ankles, and elbows especially, looking for areas of skin that seem tender, chafed, pink or red, and are slightly warm to the touch. If you find a suspicious-looking spot, press it with your fingers. If it is an incipient ulcer, the redness will vanish when you push down, then immediately reappear when the pressure is relieved. If the trouble spot becomes dark blue or purple and stops responding to the push test, it may already be too late. Watch it closely.

- If you identify a potential bedsore, stroke the area and rub it gently with a skin ointment. Rubbing will bring blood to the trouble spot and help prevent further deterioration.

- Be certain that the sick person's mattress is firm and that it has no protruding bumps or ridges. In general, a hard sleeping surface that distributes a person's weight is a better preventive against bedsores than a soft, spongy model.

- Be wary of heavy blankets. Their extra weight can bring pressure to problem areas and produce friction. Articles of clothing that rub, bind, or irritate the skin are taboo.

- Sheepskin or chamois underblankets will help absorb sweat, a major contributor to bedsores. Sheepskin will also supply a particularly soft, loving surface to lie on day after day, and though there is no scientific proof to back it up, popular wisdom has it that sheepskin blankets improve the quality of a person's sleep as well. Animal skin blankets of any kind should always be hand-washed and air-dried.

- Bedsores are serious, and their care should always be supervised by a physician. As soon as a break in the skin occurs, infection tends to set in quickly, and the opening can become violently inflamed. A doctor may require that a special blanket frame (called a bed cradle) be erected over the person's sleeping area so that friction between the blanket and the sore is minimized. The doctor may also suggest that a therapeutic mattress be used to relieve pressure on the problem areas. Continual exposure of the sore to sunlight will also help.

- Demented persons in different stages of debilitation have different statistical chances for developing bedsores. One key to prevention is the identification of persons who are particularly at risk. In 1962 the Norton scale (Table 4.1) was devised to determine this factor, and it is widely used today.

Foot Care.   Feet can easily become too sweaty or too dry, depending on the climate and on the amount of time they are exposed to circulating air. Since the person's feet are either wedged inside shoes or, for the bedridden, sequestered under the covers, they can quickly become a favorite haunt of dirt and bacteria. For this reason their maintenance should not be overlooked. Here are a few tips:

- Clip toenails every two or three weeks. Keep them short but not dangerously near the quick. Ingrown nails are excruciating and can easily become infected. When clipping, cut straight across the top of the nail and square off the corners. Never cut the nail lower than a fourth of an inch below the tip of the toe.

- If a person's feet perspire a great deal and are easily chafed, cotton socks will absorb irritating moisture. When feasible, allow persons to walk barefoot for at least an hour a day, and make sure their feet are exposed daily to a few minutes of direct sun. If sweating continues to be a problem, place a wad of cotton, gauze, or lamb's wool between the person's toes. This will absorb moisture and cut down on friction. Picking at the wadding can be discouraged by

TABLE 4.1   THE NORTON SCALE

Physical Condition		Mental State		Activity		Mobility		Incontinence	
Good	(4)	Alert	(4)	Ambulant	(4)	Full	(4)	Not	(4)
Fair	(3)	Apathetic	(3)	Walks with Help	(3)	Slightly Limited	(3)	Occasionally	(3)
Poor	(2)	Confused	(2)	Chairbound	(2)	Very Limited	(2)	Usually Urinary	(2)
Very bad	(1)	Stuporous	(1)	Bedfast	(1)	Immobile	(1)	Both Bowel and Bladder	(1)

A score of 14 or below indicates that a person is at risk for developing pressure sores.

Source: L. A. Goldstone and J. Goldstone, "The Norton Score: An Early Warning of Pressure Sores?" *Journal of Advanced Nursing,* 7 (1982), 419–426.

Quoted in Gurland, Barry, and Barrett, Virginia, *Special Skin Care Problems of the Incontinent Elderly and Their Health Care Providers,* Center for Geriatrics, Gerontology and Long-Term Care, Columbia University, Faculty of Medicine, p. 2 (published under a grant from The Procter & Gamble Company, 1987).

securing the material to the toes with a few strips of surgical adhesive tape.

- Avoid shoes that cramp or rub, especially in the toe areas. Panty hose and tight socks can produce foot irritation and may sometimes contribute to ingrown toenails. Avoid both.

- Periodically soak the person's feet in a solution of warm water and epsom salts. Water softens the skin, refreshes the feet, and removes residues of dead skin. Afterward, dry the feet well and rub them down with skin lotion. Then dust between the toes with baby powder.

Hair.   Morale and hygiene will both get a lift if a person's hair is combed several times a day and washed whenever it becomes matted or greasy. Persons in the early stages of dementia will usually be able to shampoo and arrange their own hair. Many women will appreciate having their hair brushed or styled now and then, and men who grew up in the years when "greasy kid stuff" was the fashion may still enjoy the scent and feel of a cream-based hair dressing.

As a rule, it is best to keep a patient's hair cut short. This way it will not easily become tangled, knotted, or sweaty, and the bits of food and debris that often find their way into long tresses can be kept at bay. Cutting a person's hair may, of course, be a struggle, especially in the later stages. Sometimes it will be necessary to steady the person's head or to hold him or her still. If the person is given to sudden, unpredictable movements, use safety scissors with rounded tips. Electric clippers, if their sound is not intimidating to the person, make the task easier and quicker.

The bedbound should, of course, also receive periodic hair washings. To wash an invalid's hair, have the person lie across the bed with his or her head hanging over the edge. Place an empty bucket beside the bed and position it directly beneath the person's head. Cover the bedsheets with a waterproof spread, drape a dry washcloth over the eyes for protection, and wedge a rolled-up towel or pillow under the neck for proper elevation. Then fill a pitcher full of warm water (being sure to test the water temperature first) and pour it slowly over the hair, letting all excess water drip into the bucket below. Apply a small amount of shampoo, massage in gingerly, and rinse several times until all soap is removed. When clean, squeeze the extra water from the hair and gently towel dry. Here are a few tips:

- If a hair dryer does not frighten the person, it will speed up the drying process considerably.
- Dry shampoos clean hair almost as well as soap and water, and they work especially well for bedbound persons.
- Don't use too much shampoo. It is not always easy to remove all the soap when a person is in the lying position, and over time soap residues will make the scalp dry and itchy.
- Baby shampoo is excellent for the job: It is mild, it does not burn the eyes, and it requires less rinsing than other shampoos.

Teeth and Dentures.   If a survey were taken of common afflictions that plague demented persons, gum disease would be a strong contender for first place. Uncared-for mouths quickly become a breeding ground for bacteria and shortly thereafter a major target for infection, with gum disease leading the list. Health care professionals do not usually check a patient's mouth, and at a certain stage the demented person may no longer be able to voice complaints. Basically this area of home care is up to the caregiver; here are some steps that can be taken to help:

- Make sure the person brushes his or her teeth after every meal. If the person cannot brush, the caregiver will have to do it.
- Make sure the sick person's diet is rich in vegetables and fruits, and hence in vitamin C, a lack of which will quickly cause gum problems. Poor nutrition in general is a major cause of gum irritation.
- Keep the person's mouth clean throughout the day. Brushing will help, as will mouthwash and rinsing after meals. Encourage the person to drink plenty of water and to eat lots of watery fruits. Also be on the alert for bad breath; it can indicate that increased oral care is needed.
- Examine the person's mouth regularly. Look for red gums, sores, tongue lesions, signs of tooth decay, and general discoloration. Especially bad for a person is to go to bed at night with a dirty mouth. During sleep persons may lie supine, and vast amounts of bacteria will collect in the back of the mouth. These accumulations can cause infection of the parotid (or salivary) glands, producing a ripe case of parotitis. You can recognize this ailment, so common among bedbound patients, by a low-grade fever and skin that is warm to the touch. Often parotitis is diagnosed as a simple cold

and aspirins are administered, with no healing effect. The whole problem can be avoided by careful oral hygiene.

- Supervise the cleaning of dentures. Use a basin of water, and, if possible, let patients scrub their own dentures. A mild soap or dentifrice should be used, and the dentures should then be rinsed in cold water.
- Periodic checks to make sure that dentures are still fitting properly can save a lot of grief down the line when the ill-fitting objects start chafing and cutting into the gums. If you have any questions about denture size and fit, a visit to the dentist's office may be in order.

Shaving. Even men in the late stages of dementia feel better when shaved; this male morale booster endures to the end. Electric shavers are, of course, easier and safer than razors and should *always* be used with persons who are prone to violent or sudden movements, or who suffer from myoclonic jerks. Do not let persons shave themselves if there is any sign of manual coordination loss or if they cannot remember the steps in the shaving process. Cologne or after-shave lotion will mask unpleasant odors and will make the person feel refreshed.

Hands and Fingernails. Like children, demented persons will put their hands into their mouths, bite on their fingers, or suck their thumbs. Constant wetting of the hands and fingers by saliva can irritate the skin and can pass potentially dangerous bacteria into the mouth. Caretakers should make certain that persons' hands are washed several times a day and that their fingernails are kept closely clipped and clean.

Sleep

One of the most difficult problems that families of AD persons face is a sick person's frequent sleeplessness. While in many instances this condition is triggered by the physiological changes that churn within the brain, other more remediable causes may also be afoot.

For example, persons who are heavily tranquilized in the evenings tend to remain sleep-laden through most of the next day as well: Come 10:00 or 11:00 that night, the person is just waking up. The sleep cycle has been reversed.

Or if sleep medication is given over a period of time, as it was with Janice M., a sixty-two-year-old cashier, the patient may suffer "paradoxical" or reverse drug effects. In Janice's case, a sedative taken for more than a month's time produced a kind of manic high, and Janice stopped sleeping almost entirely. A physician had to be called in, and another round of sedatives and tranquilizers was prescribed, then another, and another. It took several months before Janice's condition could be stabilized, and by that time sleep deprivation had taken its toll: Soon afterward she became unmanageable at home and had to be permanently institutionalized.

A common method for returning a patient to a regular sleep cycle is to reduce sedative dosage so that the person is less sleepy during the day and increasingly fatigued at night. In some cases, simply taking a person off sedatives entirely and tiring them out with natural methods will do the trick. Exercise, a full day of activities, trips to a respite center, walks, visits, no caffeine, a high-carbohydrate diet at night, a hot bath, and three 500-mg tryptophan pills before bed can all help.

At other times, both natural means and moderate medication will fail to do the job. Somehow the brain centers that trigger slumber simply go haywire, and like it or not, the person is up and pacing frantically most of the night. Professionals refer to this situation as the "sundowning syndrome."

Reg: During the day Mom was quiet as a mouse. She hardly said or did anything other than play with an old fox fur she loved and mutter to herself. Come the evening she would become a whirlwind. She would pace the room. She would rattle the window frame and bang on the walls. She would tear the covers off her bed. She would move the chairs around. She would bite the woodwork—all that kind of thing. This went on every night and created a terrible racket in our house. At one point we tried putting restraints on Mom at night, but that was a backfire for us. She just sat there and bellowed and rattled the chair till it drove us bonkers. Luckily, this was just a stage. The midnight prowling didn't last but about eight or nine months. One thing did help. That was to take her out for a walk after dinner, just around the time when she started getting nuts. That calmed her and made her nights better.

There is not always a lot you can do about sundowning, short of total narcotic stupefaction, a condition that you will of course want to avoid. Indeed, if persons are irrevocably locked into sundowning behavior and if space permits, you may have to leave them to their own devices, allowing them to pace, wander, walk about, mutter, slam, and bang. But let them do it alone, in their own room. The trick now, if you are to stay sane while all this is happening, is to get enough sleep yourself.

This can be accomplished in several ways. Try locking the person in for the night and removing yourself to the opposite end of the house or apartment. If your space is small and the person's sleeping area is nearby, try earplugs. Morton R. helped shut out the noise of his pacing wife by adding soundproofing materials to the walls and door of her room. One man discovered that a TV set left on at night in his wife's room had a soporific effect, even though she never actually watched it. Some people find that going into the person's room and conversing quietly for a few minutes in a soothing voice has a calming effect. In some instances the only answer is heavy sedation.

Whatever methods you come up with for assuring yourself of a quiet night, be certain that you do not remain passive before the dilemma. Sleep is crucial. Without it you will become a zombie at work and a tyrant at home. Social workers, nurses, and home aides often have good suggestions for solving this upsetting but common problem, as do other caregivers one meets at self-help groups. The discussion of wandering in Chapter 7 goes into this question in depth.

5

Improving Communication with Demented Persons

One of the most forlorn sights that family members can witness during the course of their caregiving stint is the gradual erosion of communication that takes place between themselves and the patient. It is difficult indeed to believe that this is the same person who was once so sensible and shrewd and simpatico, or, conversely, whose angry and dominating personality kept people continually worried and under control. This same personality is now helpless and in a stage of void. All that passion and force, all that vice and virtue is seeping out day by day, and in its place silence and coldness have come, unemotive affect and an unaware brain. "It's as if we were watching Grandma slowly freezing in a block of ice," an articulate caregiver named Rachel L. described it.

> The outer part of her seemed to freeze first. Her facial expressions got hard and fixed like a beeswax mask. She stopped smiling. She didn't even change her expression when she ate. It got so she would speak in this slow, robotlike voice which was almost unhuman. It just wasn't Grandma here anymore. Then the cold moved more inward until it reached her heart and soul, and then she froze over completely. Pretty soon everything about her was encased. She just couldn't hear or see or care anymore.

Without communication between giver and receiver, nothing is left over to connect with and to exchange. The human part is vanished, and only a shell of blood and brains is left behind. The goal of quality caregiving, therefore, should clearly be to prolong communication between patient and caregiver for as long a time as one can, and on as high a level as possible.

Is this goal achievable? Are there really methods that can be used to help the patient relate to others in a better way and for a longer period of time?

Many persons believe there are. As new research data become available and as an ever-increasing number of hours are logged with AD patients, many health care professionals believe that steps can be taken both to heighten the quality of verbal exchange—though clinically this is still not a certainty—to prolong the amount of time during which the patient remains capable of effective communication.

Certainly there are those who would argue with this idea, insisting that the process of a patient's cognitive decline is analogous to a wind-up mechanism that runs down according to a preprogrammed schedule and that any attempt that caretakers might make to impede its progress is a waste of time. Others, however, believe that the rate at which this decline advances depends not only on a cruel biological clock but on the quality of the patient's environment and personal interactions as well. Although nothing we can do will ultimately prevent the decline, they report, things can be done to slow it down.

Over the past few years, therefore, many specialists in psychology, occupational therapy, speech therapy, dance and art therapy, and related fields have worked out a number of ingenious methods for improving communication between caregiver and demented patient. Prominent among professionals who are presently pioneering in this brave new field is a language pathologist, Dr. Lynne H. Clark. An associate of the Brookdale Center and program director of the Communication Sciences program at Hunter College in New York, Dr. Clark has spent the past several years observing hundreds of Alzheimer's patients, both on a personal level and in group situations. During this time she has come to believe that with adequate training, not only can caregivers be taught to communicate in a more direct and effective way with demented patients, but also that the quality of the communicative methods themselves will produce a sustaining effect on patients' well-being, perhaps even helping them maintain their present level of communication function for longer periods of time. The material that follows is based on current theories in speech-language pathology and on Dr. Clark's most recent work with dementia.

Stages of Communication Loss

Though fully aware of the fact that dividing Alzheimer's disease into stages is an arbitrary tool at best and one that is subject to both exception and ambiguity, Dr. Clark has repeatedly observed that demented persons do tend to pass through three main levels of linguistic and communicative deterioration, designated mild, moderate, and severe, and that there are two transitional stages between these principal levels as well, the "moderate to severe" (which precedes the severe) and a final or "marked" stage that comes at the end.

At each level, patients tend to show specific clinical changes, both in their capacity to deal with the world and in their ever-lessening ability to speak their minds and express their feelings. Gaining knowledge of what to expect at each stage, and how to handle the specific problems and contingencies indigenous to each will thus be of substantial help to caregivers as their patients' conditions develop. We shall describe these stages and give guidelines for self-help and home care. You will learn the following things:

1. How to recognize the stages of communicative decline that the patient passes through during the course of Alzheimer's disease
2. How to anticipate and identify the clinical changes that accompany the significant stages
3. Practical suggestions for maximizing rapport with patients and devising appropriate communication strategies at each level of cognitive impairment
4. Methods for enhancing both the patient's well-being and the caregiver's peace of mind through improved verbal and nonverbal interactions

The first of the five stages is known as the "borderline to mild" stage. It is not always easy to identify.

Stage One: Borderline to Mild

Communication Goals

Identify the problems and, with medical help, make sure they are actually caused by a progressive dementia. Try to keep the patient's social exchanges as close to normal as possible. Supply patients with basic methods for dealing with linguistic and semantic losses.

Clinical Changes You Can Expect to See

The earliest signs of dementia, as we have already seen, may not be easy to tell apart from the normal, everyday symptoms of aging. Short-term memory deficits harass both the normal patient and the afflicted one, as does a reduced ability to concentrate or a slacking off of efficiency on the job. What sets demented patients off from the normal, if we can capsulize the difference in a phrase, is that these symptoms occur with greater frequency and more profound intensity in demented persons than in normal persons. The following signs may also be tip-offs.

During the Course of a Conversation, Patients in the Mild Stage of Dementia May Tend to Show Delayed Response Between Each Word and Sentence.   Mom is usually sharp as a tack. It's just that during the past several months you've noticed that several prolonged moments elapse from the time you address her to the moment she replies. If this delay is already typical of this person, as it sometimes is, fine. But if not, the change may be worth noting. Long, unusual pauses between words and sentences are also a possible sign, but again, only if it is atypical.

Hints and suggestions: Patients in the mild stages of dementia can usually find the word they are looking for. They may simply have to struggle for it a bit harder than usual. If the patient does start to respond with a delayed reply, identify the problem, then give the patient more time to get the words out.

When Patients Cannot Think of the Exact Word, They Will Often Use a Circumlocution.   A patient who cannot think of the word for hat or pancake or cane will get the meaning across in some other way, using indirect or roundabout language in place of a precise noun. Instead of saying, "Can you help me find my razor?" Jed R. told his wife: "I'm looking for that sharp thing that I shave with, honey. Have you seen it?" Later that day Jed was playing with his grandson's puppy. Instead of telling his wife that the dog needed more water, he said: "Honey, this little thing's thirsty. I think he needs more stuff in the bowl."

Hints and suggestions: Circumlocution is a good technique for the patient and should be encouraged. It's a sign that he or she is attempting to self-medicate, as it were, to compensate for the loss of communicative skills with an alternate method that is almost as good. Encourage these attempts. If the patient is receptive to the idea, suggest ways of using circumlocution in everyday speech.

Patients Will Digress for a Short Time from the Topic at Hand.   Let us eavesdrop on Eva's dialogue with her daughter. Eva was recently diagnosed as having some variety of progressive dementia, though which kind is not yet certain:

Eva:	I want to go to the store this afternoon, dear. I need some things.
Eva's daughter:	What kinds of things, Mother?
Eva:	Well . . . some tissue to clean my glasses. They've gotten very dirty with all this dust. It's gotten into my nose and eyes badly today. I've sneezed about a hundred times. Gets this way every spring. The air's filled with the pollen, don't you know. The wind blows it around all over the place. Oh yes, and I also need some soap, and some thumbtacks, and . . .

Hints and suggestions: In the beginning stages of dementia, a patient's ability to communicate will still be quite functional. Patients may ramble a bit during conversation, but they will usually return to the subject at hand without prompting. At this stage you need only sit tight and let them do the correcting for themselves. If they do not eventually get back on track after a digression, wait for the right opportunity, then gently break into the conversation with such nonintrusive phrases as "Weren't you going to tell me about . . ." or "I think you were just saying that . . ."

Patients Will Tend to Make Evaluative and Personalized Statements at the Expense of Objective Fact. A common testing procedure used by speech-language pathologists is to show patients a picture and ask them to explain what is going on. For example, a typical test picture might show a large and busy kitchen. A young boy is standing on a stool, reaching for a cookie jar, and the stool is about to tip. Nearby a woman is standing drying dishes, but the water in the sink is overflowing. The picture, in other words, depicts a dramatic and attention-getting scene with an easily recognized narrative line and plenty of interesting action.

When normal younger persons are asked to describe this or pictures like it, they report the action in impartial terms without bringing in their own personal experience: for example, "A boy is standing on a stool trying to reach for some cookies. The stool is tipping over. There's a woman nearby—it looks like his mother—and she's washing the dishes, but the sink is running over."

A person in the early stages of dementia will be less inclined to recite the circumstantial facts of the event and more likely to personalize the images. For example, when Norma S., a seventy-one-year-old mother of five children was shown the picture, her description went something like this:

> *Norma:* Gee, that woman looks something like my Aunt Grace used to look when she cooked in the kitchen. That was almost sixty years ago now. She'd always make such a mess with the water at the sink. The boy is like Tad was at that age. Look at how he stands, with the same bend to his back and all. I guess we'd all be filling our bellies if the cookie jar was near. . . .

Hints and suggestions: Personalizing unrelated events rather than reporting them objectively can be an early sign of cognitive impairment. Keep an eye out for it. However, remember that many normal elderly persons also tend to personalize objective facts with some frequency.

Patients Will Often Correct Their Verbal Communication Errors. Patients at this stage may be acutely aware of their verbal slips and miscommunications. They will try to hide their mistakes by joking about them ("Can't even remember a simple word like *birthday*—I must be getting senile!"), changing the subject, glossing over the inaccuracy, or correcting the mistake quickly and going on.

Hints and suggestions: Never embarrass or challenge elderly persons when and if they attempt to hide their mistakes. Allow them the pretense and move on. Mockery can cause patients to turn inward and close down.

Further Suggestions for Enhancing Communication in the Mild Stage of Dementia

1. Get patients' attention before speaking to them. Touching them on the arm or shoulder will focus their eyes and ears on you. If a person does not care to be touched—some AD patients do not—address the person in a louder than usual voice before speaking. Speak only when you are visible to the person.

2. Establish eye contact and maintain it throughout the conversation. Eye contact will serve as a hook to keep the patient's attention fixed on your words and gestures. If possible, situate yourself at the same positional level as the patient: If he or she is sitting, sit; if standing, stand. Four to six feet apart is the perfect distance for carrying on a comfortable conversation. Always face the listener when you are speaking so that he or she can benefit from the visual cues of facial expression and mouth movements.

3. Speak slowly and allow patients plenty of time to respond. It may sometimes be necessary to say a sentence twice or to repeat it again

slowly and distinctly. Take twice as long to form your words as you usually do, and make the effort to shape your words very clearly. Comprehension problems at this stage are related specifically to memory, length of message, attention, and a slowed ability to process auditory and visual information. Speaking slowly and carefully will help in all four areas.

4. Because AD patients are easily distracted and confused, the quieter and simpler the environment, the better able a patient will be to interact freely. This means keeping the radio low, turning down record players, turning off the TV. Patients do best in a one-to-one conversational situation, and early in the game many elderly sufferers lose their ability to converse with several people in the same room. One reason for this decline is that ambient sights and sounds that we take for granted and which our senses automatically censor are no longer so easily filtered out by the demented person. Harry R., for instance, a patient in the moderately severe stage, was placed in a nursing home. Whenever his brother and sister visited him, Harry met them in the downstairs lobby. Unfortunately, the house intercom system was designed to broadcast throughout the whole building, the lobby included, and though Harry had heard similar sounds a hundred times before, whenever a voice came booming over the PA, he leaped up from his chair and started looking around, thinking he was being addressed by a doctor or a nurse. Harry had lost the normal ability to isolate conversational voices from the myriad sounds that surrounded him.

5. Speak simply and remain on one topic at a time. Do not assume that persons can follow rapid conversational transitions. They cannot. Avoid sudden shifts in topics. If the subject is changed, inform the listener, "We are talking about such-and-such right now."

6. If the listener has repeated difficulty understanding a particular word or phrase, find a different way of saying it rather than repeating the original words over and over again.

7. Avoid speaking baby talk. No one likes to be infantilized, especially demented patients in the early stages of the disease who are already in the process of becoming as dependent as children.

8. Respond with empathy to the person's expressed feelings. Keep your voice tone warm and supportive. Persons will respond less to what you say and more to the way you say it.

9. Don't take it personally if the sick person forgets important or intimate facts concerning your relationship. Birthdays, anniversaries, important moments you have shared in the past are still a vivid part of

your own memory bank; but chances are that the person's weakened mind has forgotten them, along with many other things. It is part of the disease. If these subjects come up in conversation and the person draws a blank, simply go on to another topic.

10. Use questions to keep the conversational ball rolling; center these questions on subjects that memory-impaired persons can easily relate to such as family matters or present-day events. Either/or questions are excellent, as are questions that trigger pleasant reminiscences. Asking patients for advice will help buoy their self-esteem. So will soliciting their opinions, ideas, and observations. Another helpful technique is to offer persons a choice between two responses: "Mom, do you think this wall color is OK for the kitchen, or is it a little too loud?" Try embedding problem-solving phrases into the conversation such as "Why do you think that. . . ?" or "Do you feel it would be good or bad if we sold the car?"

11. Move in an unhurried manner and use body language that conveys security and empathy. Long after persons have lost their mental acuity, they will read your expressions and gestures like a book.

12. Learn the limits of a person's attention span and do not exceed it during conversation. Short, quiet rest periods between speaking efforts will be welcomed by caregiver and patient alike. Keep in mind that all of us hear better and understand better when we are free of fatigue, illness, and distraction.

13. When initiating a conversation, begin by introducing the topic to be discussed. Don't be shy about this; announce the subject clearly and with gusto: "Bill, I want to tell you about Linda's trip to Brazil." "OK, Mom, let's talk about the time we all went fishing on the dock at Beaver Lake." Go from the general to the specific; start with an overview, then fill in the details. This technique will help persons mentally organize information, and their responses will be accordingly appropriate.

14. Break down complex thoughts into simple phrases. Avoid long, winding sentences and third person pronouns; for example: "Dad, last night Judith and I felt like eating out because Judith didn't want to cook, so we went over to Louie's and ordered some of your favorite dishes, veal parmesan—remember, the kind with the cheese on it and the red sauce?" It would be better to break such narratives down into simple questions and declarative sentences: "Dad, last night Judith and I went out to dinner. Judith was tired. Judith didn't want to cook. So we went to one of your favorite restaurants in the neighborhood. The restaurant called Louie's. Judith and I ordered veal parmesan at Louie's. Remember,

that's the veal dish you like so much? The dish with cheese and that delicious red sauce on it? We thought of you while we ate it."

15. When persons digress, bring them back to the topic at hand by asking pertinent questions. Avoid the confrontational ("Come on, Mom, you're getting off the subject again!"). Instead, ask a question that relates to what the person was speaking about before the digression occurred, such as: "About what you were just saying, Dad—do you think you'll need that new air filter or not?" or "What were you telling me about mixing the chocolate and the raisins before? That sounded delicious."

16. Avoid talking for other people and filling in their omitted words. Demented persons are aware of their communication problems at this point and prefer not to have their difficulties highlighted. If possible, give speakers room to finish all sentences on their own. Allow them time to think of words they search for; they will eventually find them. Where it is absolutely necessary to help out, try indirect, nonconfrontational methods. Point to the actual object being searched for. Use such phrases as "Maybe it's an *X* you want, Pete." Instead of shouting "cup!" when Grandmother can't get the word out, go to the cabinet, point to a cup, and ask if this is what she needs. This approach cuts down on frustration and improves relationships between everyone.

17. Phrase sentences in the present tenses. Many of us have a tendency to use the passive voice rather than active when speaking. We say, "The letter was written by the secretary." Such constructions are easily understood by normal persons, but they can drive a demented patient into a paroxysm of confusion. Avoid such potential entanglements by speaking in the simple present or simple past tense: "The secretary writes the letter" or "The secretary wrote the letter."

Stage Two: Moderate

Communication Goals

Goals at this stage include keeping the present level of verbal ability intact for as long as possible and helping speakers learn ways to compensate for impaired communication. Caregivers should strive to make afflicted persons feel that they can still communicate successfully without feeling embarrassed or frustrated.

Clinical Changes You Can Expect to See

Be prepared to see a marked reduction in factual knowledge and in individuals' abilities to perform complex daily tasks such as shopping for food or reading a book. Persons may be unable to travel alone to unfamiliar places; they may begin voluntarily to withdraw from social encounters.

True, many individuals continue to communicate effectively in familiar settings. But difficulties of expression and comprehension will increase in strange or confusing situations. Meanwhile, while these declines are taking place, persons may also assert that nothing is wrong with them, that everything is just fine. "I'm all right, Jack" is the patient's predominant line at this stage of the illness. Other communication changes that mark the moderate stage include the following:

When Persons Forget a Word, They Will Substitute a Closely Related Word. As dementia progresses, the types of word loss change too. In the milder stages, circumlocution is applied to offset word retrieval difficulties. At the moderate level, persons use terms that are *related* to the forgotten word but are not alike in meaning. These words may be associationally or emotionally linked. They may even be opposites. When Hattie wanted someone to pass the sugar, she asked for the salt instead. When Lawrence saw a dog, he called it a cat. Whenever Laverne rode up in the elevator, she spoke of it as the stairs. Ben referred to the TV as the hi-fi. Charlie said he wanted to take a drive "in the road"; he meant the car. Technically speaking, this tendency is referred to as semantic paraphrasia.

Hints and suggestions: You can penetrate to the meaning of these off-target words by interpreting them within the context of the situation. If your husband is eating french fries and tells you to pass the sugar, you know he means the salt. If Mom asks to have the roof closed and the window is open, the meaning is clear. The caregiver, in other words, learns to interpret and decipher. He or she strains to read between the jumbled lines, to find the hidden meanings behind the word play, to apply situational logic to the person's sometimes illogical requests.

If individuals continue to have trouble pinpointing a specific word, you can help them find it by using a number of techniques, including these:

- In circumstances where it is impossible to tell what persons are asking for, offer them a choice: "Do you want the salt" (pointing to the salt) "or the sugar?" (pointing to the sugar). "Do you want a pencil? A pen? Some paper?"
- Ask persons to think of a word that is *like* the one they cannot remember. Go down a list. Jeannie was asking for something to

drink. Her nurse recited several choices: "Do you want orange juice?" "No." "Water?" "I don't like water." "Milk?" "No." "Soda?" "Yes, that's what I want. Soda pop."

- Some persons find it helpful to keep lists of important words in their pocket and to refer to these as needed. Work with the person to collect and write down words they will need in their day-to-day activities.

- Ask your loved one to use gestures when expressing needs. If Aunt Lucille is searching for a pen, she can mimic writing. If Grandfather is looking for a magazine, he will hold his hands in front of his face as if reading.

- Ask persons to describe the object they are speaking of. Then ask direct questions about it: What is the object made of? How big is it? In what part of the house might it be found? What is it used for?

Demented Persons May Use Clichés and Excuses to Cover Up Their Disabilities.   When Marie went to the doctor's office for a physical exam, the doctor asked her how she was feeling. "Oh, fine," she replied. "How's your heart? Any problems?" asked the doctor. "Never felt better," Marie answered. "But how are *you*, Doctor Rolfe?" she then wanted to know. "You're looking your usual handsome self today."

In other words, instead of revealing that she wasn't sure what her "heart" actually was and instead of admitting that she had some *very* big problems, Marie shifted the point of attention away from herself and onto the other person. "If I hadn't known Marie was suffering from Alzheimer's disease," Dr. Rolfe said later, "I would honestly have thought she was fine."

Hints and suggestions: Although persons in the moderate stage lose some grip on the formal meaning of words, they still maintain a firm hold on the social deployment of language, using charm and polite disclaimers to get around the communicative problems at hand. This can be a good tool and should be encouraged. It will help persons feel good about themselves for a long time to come. At the same time, don't let it fool *you*. It would be folly to confront ailing persons about their "hypocrisy," but there is no cause for you to be taken in by such artful deceptions and to develop false hopes.

Persons May Abruptly Digress from the Topic of Conversation and Not Return to It Unless Prompted.   In the mild stages of dementia, persons catch themselves going off the subject and quickly return. In the moderate stage, this ability begins to fade. Speakers drift off, never to reestablish their chain of thought; sometimes they start to free-associate; occasionally they talk in gibberish.

Hints and suggestions: At this point you must intervene and pull the person back to the subject at hand. Do it politely and subtly: "What were you saying before, Dad?" "Let's get back to what we were talking about a minute ago, Nancy. You were saying some interesting things." Whatever you do and however you do it, always help the afflicted person maintain his or her self-respect.

Patients May Begin to Withdraw and May Stop Initiating Conversations. During the late moderate stage, AD sufferers may begin to experience motor and coordination problems. Coupled with increased cognitive disorders, these physical and mental losses can tip the stress balance in a negative way, triggering a dramatic increase in social withdrawal.

Hints and suggestions: Withdrawal can be controlled at this stage, but you will have to work at it. One of the best ways to keep moderately severe persons socially involved is to capture their attention on a tactile, sensory level. For example, eighty-one-year-old Marjorie was an excellent seamstress before she developed dementia. So her caregiver, a young woman named Leslie who has been trained in physical therapy, comes to Marjorie's room each day carrying a small packet of fabrics, thread, beads, sequins, and assorted sewing equipment. Leslie starts off by asking Marjorie, who at this point is at the moderately severe stage, which fabrics she finds pretty, which color thread she prefers, and so forth. Since Marjorie's hands remain well coordinated, she is able to sew for a few minutes every day under Leslie's supervision. Soon, however, Marjorie's concentration wanes, and then Leslie encourages her to play with the fabric, to stroke it, finger it, fold it into neat, handkerchieflike packets.

Here is another example: Don loved sports before he developed dementia. Now when Don's son Robert visits, he brings a scrapbook full of old sports clippings. Since Don is approaching the severe stage and can no longer turn pages, his son does it for him. The two men sit together in the living room and study the pictures, sometimes for long periods of time. Given Don's present level of impairment, he is often not sure what he is looking at even when his son provides the narrative. But Don enjoys these sessions nonetheless, this everyone in the family is sure of, and he frequently tries to prolong the experience. Sometimes he will point to a picture and laugh happily.

Use props and mementos. Bring a set of party napkins and ask Mother which she thinks would be appreciated at tonight's dinner party. Use personal cues that revive past remembering. A beloved jewelry box may do the trick, or a favorite fountain pen, a baseball, a photograph, some beads, a figurine, a typewriter, a trowel and potting soil—whatever triggers happy recollections. The secret of using props to their fullest advantage is to introduce positive emotional associations that make persons feel connected once again to the tactile and visual pleasures of life.

Note that midway through the moderate stage, afflicted persons may no longer be capable of back-and-forth conversation, and trying to force such dialogue can quickly become an exercise in futility. The truth is that patients at this stage are simply not responsive to such conventional icebreakers as "How are you today, Boyd?" or "Hey, you're looking great, Ruth." In other words, don't assume that because you speak, AD sufferers will speak back. They may not. Their sense of social propriety is eroded. They may be depressed or lethargic or simply incapable of conversation. Again, props that trigger recall will help. So will questions that evoke reminiscence, that solicit opinions or seek advice, that plug into memories that feel good and inspire happy recollections.

Persons May Ask You to Repeat Your Sentence Several Times Before They Understand What You Are Saying.   Here's another sign that comprehension is fading. Sentences that sound clear and explicit to a normal ear may reverberate like gobbledygook in the AD patient's mind. The person may ask you several times or more to repeat the most simple phrases:

"How are you feeling today, Joyce?"

"What?"

"How are you today?"

"Uhhh?"

"How . . . are . . . you . . . today, . . . Joyce?"

(After a long pause) "What?"

Hints and suggestions: Be patient. When you repeat your sentences, say them slowly and enunciate every word. Exaggerate your mouth movements: Make large *o*'s and *m*'s and *v*'s with your lips as you speak. Accompany your words with expressive gestures and expressions.

Patients Will Have Difficulty Drawing Logical Inferences and Filling In Meaning Gaps.   When normal persons converse, they take certain information for granted. If I have a headache, I say, "My head hurts." I don't have to tell listeners what my head is, where it is located, or what it is used for. But this is not so with demented patients. At a certain stage you will have to stop taking *anything* for granted. You will have to be as precise and obvious in your language as possible; even the most trifling detail counts if you wish to communicate effectively.

Hints and suggestions: When speaking with demented persons, break down your sentences into discrete packets of information, and make no assumptions. Instead of telling your loved one that you are "going to the store," say something like this: "Mother, we have no more bananas or milk. I am going to drive the car to the food store now. I will shop there for the bananas and milk. I'll return here in an hour or so. Janet will be here with you while I'm gone."

Persons Will Have Trouble Following Directions and Performing Complex Daily Tasks; They Must Be Verbally Coached.   Elderly persons in the moderate stage of dementia begin to have real problems with household chores and with keeping themselves clean. At this stage they are capable of following one- or two-step directions but not much more. You will have to help.

Hints and suggestions: Break tasks down into short steps, and accompany your instructions with visual demonstrations. When Minnie's sister helps Minnie dress each morning, no longer can she simply place a few articles of clothing on the bed and tell Minnie to get dressed. Now she must talk her sister through the process a step at a time. First, she tells Minnie to remove her nightgown, and if help is needed, she gives it. She tells Minnie to fold the nightgown, shows her which drawer to put it in, and reminds her to close the drawer. Then together they pick out Minnie's clothes for the day. First the undergarments. If Minnie forgets how to put them on, her sister pantomimes the process. Then the skirt, the bra, the blouse. With each article of clothing, Minnie's sister is there for Minnie, explaining what to do if help is needed and watching carefully if it is not.

Further Suggestions for Enhancing Communication in the Moderate Stage of Dementia

1. Address individuals in a louder tone than usual and by name. If they are disoriented, remind them of their name, where they are, and the names of other family members.

2. Avoid using abstract or nonspecific words with moderately im-

paired persons. Do not say, "Do you want this?" Say, "Do you want this washcloth?" Minimize abstract questions such as "Are you feeling cold?" Say instead, "Do you want me to put this extra blanket over your legs?"

3. When persons use incorrect words and you are unsure of what they are asking, offer them a choice. For instance, say, "Do you want the coffee or the tea, Dad?" "Is it the leg that's hurting you or the arm?" Tell persons you do not know what they are talking about only as a last resort.

4. Communicate one idea at a time, using common words and friendly, emotive gestures. Avoid intricate or complex verbal constructions. Describe events and ideas in logical order, keeping topics familiar, relevant, and personal. Politics and the weather report do not often capture a demented person's attention.

5. Never change the subject abruptly. AD sufferers will not be able to follow the sudden shift and may become frustrated. When the conversation does take a sudden turn, clue listeners in: "Dad we're talking about how Donna won that blue ribbon at the horse show. Remember what a good horseback rider she is?"

6. Establish a basic vocabulary of the same words and the same phrases and use them every day. Try not to introduce new words or unusual phrases into your conversation. Also, avoid slang. If you tell a person to "step on it" or "throw on your coat," they may take you literally, with disastrous consequences.

7. Listen actively to what individuals are saying. Voice inflections, expressions, and physical gestures may tell you a good deal more about what's going on inside than actual words.

8. If persons lose their train of thought, you can sometimes bring them back to the subject by repeating the last sentence they have just said.

9. Provide constant encouragement and tireless praise. Demented persons tend to overlook their successes at communication and to stress their lapses. Remind them frequently of how well they have done and how well they are doing now. This can really help, even if the persons do not directly acknowledge your praise.

10. Structure your verbal and nonverbal communications so that they match an individual's present level of comprehension and cognitive ability.

11. When giving instructions, reinforce them by writing them down and posting them in a conspicuous place. Written messages like "Drink Your Water" or "Wash Your Hands" can often be understood, even by

patients in relatively advanced levels of dementia. Write in large, bold printed letters—script may be difficult to read.

12. If persons are having difficulty getting started at a particular physical task, help them out. If they want to comb their hair, move their hand through the combing motion several times. After a few tries, they will usually remember how it is done.

13. Avoid using third-person pronouns like *he, it,* or *they.* AD sufferers will probably not know whom or what you are referring to. Cite all persons and objects by name. Don't say, "He is coming in a minute." Say, "Robert is coming in a minute, Dad." Don't say, "Pick it up." Say, "Pick up the tray, Mom."

Stage Three: Moderate to Severe

Communication Goals

Persons at this stage are usually capable of communicating and interacting only on the most basic levels. Caregivers' goals include encouraging any skills that are still intact, devising new and effective communication methods suited to patients' present level of understanding, and helping persons salvage whatever self-awareness and autonomy remains.

Clinical Changes You Can Expect to See

Persons will begin to experience noticeable motor difficulties. They will be severely limited in their capacity to make needs known and will require assistance when dressing and bathing. Specific changes to look for at this stage include the following:

Use of Words Becomes Increasingly Imprecise.   Instead of "dog," persons ask about "that animal." Instead of an "apple," they request a piece of "food." Instead of "television set," they want to watch "pictures." Persons who previously tended to mix up or forget their nouns now start slipping on their verbs as well. They forget the word *write* and use *draw* instead, they substitute *run* for *drive* or *look* for *read.*

Hints and suggestions: Play the elimination game. If a person is asking for a certain food but can't think of its name, give choices. "Do you want some fruit? Like an apple? An orange? A banana? Do you want something to drink? Juice? Coffee?" Though persons cannot verbalize their needs precisely at this stage, they still know what they want and will usually respond affirmatively when you hit the nail on the head.

Expressive Vocabulary Becomes Markedly Reduced. Not only do demented persons now say less, but they express what they do say in more primitive terms. Vocabulary shrinks. Sentence structures become less complex and complete. Thoughts and feelings are presented in the most fundamental terms.

Hints and suggestions: Keep the voice exercised in an enjoyable way by singing familiar songs together. Easily recalled children's songs such as "Row, Row, Row Your Boat" or "I've Been Working on the Railroad" will do, though any tunes persons like are fine. Frequent singing not only gives the speaking and swallowing muscles a workout but jogs word memory as well.

Persons Will Have Difficulty Recognizing Simple Words. Words such as *brush, faucet,* or *wastebasket* may now bring silent stares of incomprehension. Whereas in the earlier stages of dementia patients had difficulty following complex thoughts but were able to comprehend ordinary vocabulary words, now they may start blanking on words as well.

Hints and suggestions: If a person cannot decipher a particular word, provide more information on its meaning. If the word *cup* draws an uncomprehending stare, explain that it is "the thing you drink from and the coffee goes into." Also of value are terms and phrases related to the forgotten word. For example, if a person is baffled by the word *notebook,* explain that it is "that *spiral* book with the *cardboard covers* and the *lines* on the *pages* where you *write* things down." All the italicized words here serve as potential cues.

Persons May Either Talk Excessively or Withdraw from Conversation Entirely. Although it is impossible to make precise correlations, we often see that individuals who tended to be reserved and introspective before they were sick become extremely silent at this stage, while those who were loquacious tend to chatter, sometimes in an obsessive and nonsensical way. Individuals who fall into this latter category may characteristically indulge in excessive detail finding and overexplanation. If, for instance, they are shown a picture that depicts two persons hugging one another in a room, they may describe every object in the room down to the most trivial detail yet miss the fact that the real subject of the picture is a couple embracing.

Hints and suggestions: To control the tendency toward extraneous detail, keep persons on track by interrupting with who, what, when, and how kinds of questions. If persons are, say, describing early life on a farm and dwell too much on descriptions of barnyard animals, you can refocus the conversation by asking questions like "Why did you like the goats so much when you were a child?" "How old were you when you first milked a cow?" "What were some of the other things you liked to do on the farm?" "Who helped you with the chores when you were young?"

Persons May Repeat the Same Word or Sound Over and Over. Word repetition begins during the moderate-to-severe stage. Patients will endlessly recite a person's name or may repeat strange, single consonant sounds like "Ca, ca, ca, ca, ca, ca, ca, ca, ca!"

Hints and suggestions: Word repetition is extremely dismaying for caregivers. Usually it is clear that patients have no control over their babbling, and asking them to quiet down seldom has an effect. Note, however, that demented persons also tend to lapse in and out of this habit and that it calms down on its own after a while. This means that when the chatter begins, caregivers can simply leave the room and return later on when it has ceased. Sometimes there is just no other choice.

Further Suggestions for Enhancing Communication in the Moderate-to-Severe Stage of Dementia

1. When conversing with demented persons, talk about what they are doing at the moment. Avoid conversations about abstract subjects, about things in the future, or about nonpersonal topics such as politics.

2. Before doing anything with or to a person, announce your intentions: "Mom, we're going to give you a bath now." "Linda, I have good news: John and Vince are here, and they want to come upstairs and visit you if they may."

3. During meals, observe how well individuals chew and swallow their food. Look for danger signs such as swallowing chunks or wads of food kept impacted in the cheeks. At some point most persons will develop feeding problems and these tend to center around mastication. If chewing becomes a problem, stop giving solids and switch to baby foods.

4. When communication problems become severe, avoid bombarding a person with too many questions and too much conversation. Stay with a few meaningful words and phrases that the person relates to and understands.

5. Even if persons have stopped talking entirely and are unaware of their environment, be careful of what you say in their vicinity. We really have no idea how much demented persons actually do or do not understand, even when in the last stages of dementia. By saying critical or

ridiculing things at the bedside, we run the risk that persons will hear and perhaps understand.

6. Observe what a person's body behavior is telling you. Often it represents a kind of silent language of its own. Facial expressions, gestures, body postures, voice sounds, movements, eye expressions, hand movements, and pointing can all be silent pleas for food, changing, turning, attention, whatever. Say aloud what you think the person needs, then ask the person to shake his or her head yes or no in response. Each person's silent language will be different. Learn it as best you can. During the last stages of dementia, nonverbal communication is often the only avenue of exchange that remains between caregiver and loved one.

Stage Four: Severe to Final Stage

Communication Goals

In the last stages of dementia, persons will be spatially and temporally disoriented and may no longer recognize loved ones and family members. Still, a majority of elderly persons will respond to nonverbal cues and, even more, to that most important tool in the caregiver's medicine bag, a loving touch. During these last stages, your goals should be to keep your loved one as comfortable as possible, to maintain whatever verbal and nonverbal communication remains between you, and to offer continual affectionate contact.

Clinical Changes You Can Expect to See

Persons will require assistance with all dressing, eating, walking, and bathroom activities, and they may no longer be capable of making their daily needs known. Bladder incontinence becomes routine, with bowel incontinence following soon after. Persons will retain only the sketchiest knowledge of their personal past, and emotional and intellectual affect will be reduced to a minimum. Expect to see disturbed sleep patterns at this time and some physical rigidity in the limbs. Specific communication changes are described below. Note, however, that at this advanced stage of Alzheimer's disease, very few suggestions can be offered, and most sufferers are institutionalized.

Persons Will Display Severe Verbal Expressive Problems.　You will not often know what they are talking about. They may babble, repeat words endlessly, talk nonsense, or indulge in *echolalia*—repeating everything back to you verbatim. When persons are capable of talking at all, moreover, their yes and no responses may be unreliable. For instance, you ask if Sally wants something to eat. She says no, but the answer is really yes. It's just that her sensation of hunger and the concept of eating are no longer clearly connected. In general, persons who are able to speak at all during the severe stage will do so with automatic phrases and one-word responses.

Hints and suggestions: Even in advanced dementia, primitive memories of reading and writing may remain intact, and sometimes a one- or two-word message printed in bold letters will get the message through. Lester, a seventy-five-year-old AD patient, had become incontinent. His family was advised by a social worker to write the word *bathroom* on a four-by-five-inch file card and hold it up to him every two or three hours. The trick worked. Lester would stare at the sign for several moments, think it over as if trying to dredge up something out of the forgotten past, then shake his head affirmatively if he had the need. Written messages can be used to determine if the person is hungry, sleepy, hot, cold, or in need of changing.

Foreign-born Patients May Revert to Their First Language. Hearing a loved one speak in a foreign language can be disconcerting, to say the least, especially if it is a language unfamiliar to the caregiver. The chances of such reversion taking place are strong if the person learned the foreign language during early childhood.

Hints and suggestions: Since the person's vocabulary is severely limited at this point, even in a foreign tongue, it may help to learn a few basic words of this language. Words such as *yes, no, hot, cold, eat,* and *bathroom* can be found in a dictionary.

Persons Fail Entirely to Understand What Is Said to Them. Cognitive systems are breaking down now in earnest. In most cases, you will simply not be able to understand what patients are trying to say, if they try to say anything at all. Knowledge of how to conduct a conversation vanishes, although persons may retain a general awareness of your presence and may respond to it in a positive or negative way.

Hints and suggestions: Long after verbal interaction has ceased, patients will understand gestures and mime. For example, if you want to tell a person that it is time to go to sleep, put both hands under your head like a pillow and make snoring sounds—nine times out of ten you will be understood. If you want the person to sit down, point to the chair and pat the seat. Or you can mimic sitting down yourself. If you want the person to eat, pantomime eating. Such play acting may be difficult at first—

Americans tend to rely less on gestures than do people of other nationalities—but when you see the fast results this method gets, you will quickly get into the swing.

Further Suggestions for Enhancing Communication in the Severe-to-Final Stage of Dementia

1. Use touch and gesture as frequently as possible, both to illustrate instructions and to communicate affection.

2. Tried and tested techniques for effective communication with persons who communicate only on a nonverbal level include the following:

- If persons are restless or walk around while you are speaking, remain in front of them and persevere until you gain their attention.
- Gently pat persons or wave to them as a sign of affection or attention getting.
- Keep your voice low, affectionate, and subdued. A high-pitched, shrill tone signals anxiety or upset and hence a physical threat. Demented persons are extremely sensitive to the emotional tones of speech.
- Use a warm smile to calm a person who has become frightened or agitated. The language of the smile endures to the end. Even blind persons can see it with their hearts.
- Use an outstretched hand to invite participation. Hold a patient's hand whenever possible. Communicate caring through the warmth and intensity of your grip.
- Put a hand on the patient's shoulder, speak his or her name, and look straight in the eyes to gain attention. Nod and smile to the person to indicate that you understand what he or she is trying to communicate. Shake hands with the person when you meet and when you are leaving.

6

Maintaining the Patient's Emotional Health

The Tombstone Syndrome

After a diagnosis of dementia has been delivered, the frequent tendency on the family's part is to assume that the patient is already beyond the pale. Known as the "tombstone syndrome," relatives may treat their newly diagnosed loved one as if he or she is already a hopeless cripple or, worse, a lifeless corpse.

Such behavior is counterproductive for all persons involved. The fact of the matter is that during the early and moderate stages of AD, many pleasures and pastimes are still available to demented persons. These pastimes do not simply keep patients occupied. They may, many professionals are now coming to believe, prolong the actual period of time in which afflicted persons remain aware and functional. This chapter profiles a number of meaningful activities that caregivers can employ to fill the patients' time and to assure that their daily life is kept intellectually rich and emotionally enlivening.

Social Life for Demented Patients

As a general rule of thumb, the social activities patients enjoyed before they became sick will continue to be enjoyed during the course of their illness. As the disease progresses, however, it becomes necessary to scale down these activities so that they fit the present level of comprehension and dexterity.

For example, Leslie had been a film agent for many years before she developed symptoms of dementia. Throughout her adult life she had enjoyed the bustle of cocktail parties and the thrill of making deals. Her favorite pastimes had been meeting with clients and carrying on phone conversations.

Leslie was lucky enough to have a loving son and daughter to look after her in her illness; her children arranged it so that in the early stages of her disease Leslie was seldom without a stream of visitors coming by her home to pay their respects. Thanks to a number of timely urgings, the phone was rarely silent, the mailbox rarely empty. When she was up to it, Leslie's children would even bring their mother to her old firm, where she would leaf through files and read the latest reviews. Leslie was especially fond of looking at the many signed photographs of motion picture personalities that still lined the walls of what had once been her private office.

Later on, when Leslie's condition became more severe and she was no longer able to converse with friends or move about on her own, her children reduced her social activities accordingly. But the pleasures they indulged her in now—videotapes of old movies, occasional phone calls from show business friends, albums full of photos and clippings—still remained centered on the people and pastimes that Leslie had enjoyed so thoroughly when she was well. Even though Leslie could no longer respond intelligently to these phone calls or film shows, it was evident from her reactions that she continued to draw pleasure from these activities and that something within her muted consciousness occasionally recognized their significance. Says Leslie's daughter of Alzheimer's patients:

> It's as if they have windows in their brains that open and shut. For a long while the windows are all shut down and no one seems to be inside looking out. Then all of a sudden one of them will pop open and for a few minutes recognition is there—Mother talks sense. She remembers who we are and who she is. She asks us things like to comb her hair or who called her today. Then the windows get shut again.

Tailoring Activities to Patient Needs

The goals caretakers set for patients' social enjoyments should take the following notions into consideration:

1. All social activities for demented patients are most readily accepted when they center on the person's previous likes, pleasures, suc-

cesses, and tastes. Do not try to introduce activities that are new or different from those that the person is accustomed to. Demented patients are not good learners, nor do they adapt well to change.

2. Activities should be geared to correspond with a patient's *current* state of comprehension and awareness. Avoid projects that are too complex, that frustrate, confuse, lower the patient's sense of mastery, or go beyond the patient's present skills.

3. When working with patients in the early stages of dementia, avoid activities that simply kill time. Persons at this stage will recognize worthless work when they see it, and they will resent being infantilized. If possible, let them choose their own entertainments. Ideally, these activities should be physically exhilarating, emotionally evocative, mentally stimulating, artistically creative, socially enriching, and/or useful to others.

4. Activities should be modified and simplified as the patient's condition declines. Keep patients under constant watch in this regard. When they seem befuddled by an activity that was previously easy to negotiate, it is time to simplify.

5. Be prepared for the fact that your ward may reject many projects you devise. Never force an activity on someone, and do not labor under the misconception that by making patients "stick with" a project you are teaching them a lesson. AD patients do not learn such lessons; discipline and moral instruction have no place here.

6. If the patient is not receptive to your current suggestions, try introducing these same ideas the next day or even an hour later. Demented patients forget from moment to moment. What they say no to at four o'clock they may eagerly accept at six.

7. Even during the later stages of dementia, patients may continue to respond to the social stimulation of fun, games, and entertainment— but only if the stimulation is simple. It should evoke pleasant associations from the past, and touch on deep, familiar joys.

The following social activities are all appropriate for demented persons in the early periods of the disease, and many can be continued into the moderate stages if modifications are made.

Home Visits from Friends

In the early stages, visitors will be welcome, especially close friends and family members. Many families, in fact, maintain a special area of the house for receiving callers. Jennifer's family set up a circle of chairs in their living room near the front door. This arrangement makes it easy for visitors to enter and leave the house, and it allows Jennifer convenient access to a sitting area when the visitors arrive. In Bob's home, visitors are shown into Bob's bedroom and are seated next to Bob's rocking chair, where he spends most of the day. During these visits, Bob's wife stands by the door. If she sees that her husband is tired or agitated from the excitement, she tells the visitors that it is time for his nap. Visitors quickly understand and take their leave.

Keep all social contacts calm and uncomplicated. One-on-one social calls are best. Visits by more than two or three persons at a time are likely to confuse patients, especially if callers all talk at the same time or frequently change the topic of conversation. To diminish confusion, caregivers can prep visitors before the visit begins, briefing them on the patient's present mental condition and pointing out the subjects the patient can and cannot comprehend. Be wary of prolonged visits and of tiring the patient with too many friendly attentions. If friends insist on bringing presents, encourage them to bring such items as food or flowers, which afford patients immediate sensory pleasure.

Note that for friends of AD patients, it can be an unpleasant experience to visit the home of a demented person and to make the efforts necessary to carry on the one-sided conversations that so often ensue. The patient no longer behaves in his or her customary social manner, and worse, the situation itself reminds visitors of something most of us wish to forget: I too will walk this way someday.

Consequently, visits from friends tend to diminish early on during the course of the person's illness, and this abandonment will produce an understandably depressing effect on all involved. Families and caregivers can, of course, fill the gap with many of the activities featured in this chapter, as well as with loving attentions. Another excellent means for promoting social life is making use of local AD day care or respite centers. Here new friendships can be quickly formed, and patients find that their physical and mental impairments are no longer the object of critical judgment. Chapter 9 goes into the subject of day care and respite centers at length.

Visiting Outside Places

In the early stages, visits to familiar people and places provide patients with emotional stimulation and a needed change of scene. Depending on the person's stamina and degree of sociability, visits can be made to the homes of friends, relatives, or, if circumstances permit, the patient's office or workplace. Since AD patients tend to be both fragile and volatile, you must keep a close eye on your charge during these calls. Any signs of agitation will signal that it is time to go home. For AD patients, even in the early stages, brief visits are usually the best visits.

Participating in Social Events

Again, depending on the patient's level of awareness and tractability, occasional outings to public places will serve as a tonic for everyone involved. Possible places to visit include these:

Restaurant	Museum
Concert	Soda fountain
Motion picture	Library
Grandchild's school	Park
Gallery	Stores
Mall	Church
Theater	Countryside

Outings in Nature

If patients spent much of their life outdoors or if they had a particular affection for nature, caregivers can see to it that they are exposed to natural settings. In a city, trips to the park will be welcomed. For country dwellers, a chair placed on the porch or on the lawn will provide fresh air and a nearness to growing things.

Even patients who are homebound or bedbound can be kept in touch with nature by surrounding them with plants, flowers, and even pets. Persons in wheelchairs can be taken out once a day and exposed to nearby flora and fauna. Flo, an elderly matron suffering from Alzheimer's for more than six years, had previously been an excellent gardener. Today she is wheelchair-bound and has not left her house for several years. Still, every afternoon her caregiver provides her with a tray of potting soil and a trowel which keeps her happily occupied for many hours of the day.

Family Gatherings

Understand that dementia almost inevitably breeds a sense of deep alienation, of separation, of being cast aside. Nothing remedies this feeling more quickly than a sense of belonging—and in many cases nothing is more pleasing than being included in family events. Whenever you can, set a place at the table during family meals for sick relatives. Let patients celebrate holidays with their families. Keep them abreast of family news. Invite them to birthdays and to special events. If possible, allow patients to come to your social gatherings or to attend your children's parties.

While some demented victims are, of course, too rowdy and restless to be included at such functions, others are manageable enough to attend; make them feel welcome. Even if the sick person sits in the corner during these affairs like a bump on a log, fine. This is a good deal better than confinement to a bed or staring at the walls. Whenever possible, *include them.*

Recreations

Hobbies

Contrary to opinion, AD patients in the early stages of their disease are still capable of pursuing a number of hobbies. Most hobbies, of course, depend on manual dexterity, and fortunately, in the first phases of dementia, motor abilities remain more or less intact. Thus such pastimes as sewing, modeling, woodworking, sketching, photography, pottery making, and model trains can be pursued as before, though now with somewhat more modest goals.

As cognitive functions begin seriously to decline, however, manual dexterity diminishes along with them. Patients soon find it difficult to figure out how a screwdriver works or what coins fit in what slots in the coin album. Tools become dangerous in inept hands. The inability to perform manual maneuvers may trigger tantrums of frustration. Finally, it seems that the hobby must be dropped entirely if peace is to reign.

Nevertheless, despite the steady erosion of cognitive functions, many hobbies can still be practiced and will continue to bring pleasure to patients if appropriate modifications are made.

1. Reduce the hobby to its simplest terms. If the patient builds models, provide only a limited selection of modeling materials: a few pieces of precut bass or balsa wood, some sandpaper, some glue. Patients who enjoyed cooking will still have fun mixing foods together or preparing extremely simple recipes such as orange juice or boiled eggs. Wood-

workers can retain a bit of the previous enjoyment if provided with several interestingly shaped blocks of wood, some nails, a plane, and a hammer. Sunday painters will usually still know what to do when given paper and colored pencils. Potters will enjoy kneading a ball of clay. Guitarists will enjoy hearing guitar music and handling their instrument.

2. If the patient can no longer control sharp or pointed tools, replace them with harmless substitutes. A wooden mallet can be used instead of a hard metal hammer. Nontoxic pastes will bind almost as well as petroleum-based glues. Oil paints can be replaced with watercolors. Crayons can be used instead of sharp-pointed pencils. A plastic shovel will dig into the ground almost as well as a metal trowel.

3. Help patients set attainable goals. While stamp collectors may no longer be able to identify foreign issues or to find a stamp's proper place in the album, they can still hinge bright new stamps onto sheets of paper and show them off. A bookbinder may have forgotten the many stages in the bookbinding process but will enjoy playing with scraps of leather, folding leaves of paper into signatures, and gluing pieces of book cloth onto cardboard boards. In other words, the tactile experience of working with hobby materials now becomes more important than the finished product. Keep hobby projects simple, and praise all results to the skies. The materials themselves will do the rest, eliciting pleasurable associations and a feeling of sensory familiarity.

4. As always, you must be tactful when dealing with a person whose cognitive abilities are fading. While some people still enjoy working with scaled-down versions of their old hobbies, others will take these reductions as yet another indication of their disintegration; they will feel put down and infantilized. For one woodworker the sight of tools will arouse pleasure and the desire to handle them. For another the same sight will bring resentment over the fact that they can no longer be skillfully used. There are no absolute rules to guide you other than to observe carefully, note how persons respond to offered activities, and remain sensitive.

Games

The rules that apply to hobbies apply to games as well. Though the AD patient will no longer be able to play bridge or chess perhaps, certain games, if appropriately scaled down, will afford patients a good deal of diversion. At certain of the Brookdale respite centers, for example, patients in the earlier stages of dementia enjoy playing a variety of games during the day, including:

Shuffleboard.   Still an old favorite. You can make a court on any flat cement surface. For a puck use a four-by-four-inch block of wood. For a stick a four-foot-long piece of one-by-two-inch lumber will do. Nail a six-inch piece of one-by-two across one end, making a T, to serve as a pusher.

Penny Pitching.   This game is especially popular at several Brookdale respite centers. Each player gets ten pennies. A shoe box is placed five or six feet away from all players, and the players are told to toss their coins into the box. "When they get one in, you shout 'Yeah! You win!' " says Wendy O'Brien, a volunteer at a New York City respite center.

> Give them a prize. Anything will do. Getting a prize makes individuals feel good somehow, even if they're not sure what they're actually winning it for. Make a big issue out of it. Call each person by name as you play: "Allen! That's very good, you got the penny into the box. You win the prize. You're a winner today!" These individuals still want to be successful. That need in a person never dies.

Balloons.   Balloons are soft, cheap, pretty, and easy to control. Hitting a balloon back and forth is fine exercise and an excellent way to stress hand-and-eye coordination. For active patients, a net can be set up and a game of balloon volleyball played.

Paper-and-Pencil Games.   Some patients will remember how to play simple children's games such as Hangman, Connect the Dots, Squares, or Tic-Tac-Toe. Other paper-and-pencil games are legion. For example, draw a picture of a face and have the patient add eyes and nose. Show pictures of various animals to patients and tell them to write the animal's name under each. Use coloring books. You will be surprised at how much fun these games can provide for some demented patients.

Puzzles.   Very simple jigsaw puzzles will still be workable by some patients. Puzzles are pretty and colorful and offer excellent mental stimulation. They will also keep some patients busy for long periods at a stretch.

Song Games.   A simple game of Sing That Tune can be fun for many elderly persons. You hum a popular tune or play it on an instrument and the person tries to sing along. Patients can also sing simple rounds like "Row, Row, Row Your Boat" or "Down by the Station." Songfests are always enjoyable, especially if the whole family is involved.

Pets

Furry creatures, with their unquestioning affections and readiness to be played with at a moment's notice, afford the kind of unambiguous love that demented persons often crave. Even sick persons who are no longer able to communicate with human beings will often retain an abiding affection for animals.

What kinds of pets are best? Puppies, as one might expect, lead the list, followed closely by kittens. Rabbits are a poor third. Then come the less intelligent creatures, the hamsters, gerbils, and white mice of the world. But do not dismiss this last group entirely. Many patients enjoy small, furry rodents as pleasant objects to handle and caress. In many cases it is the pure physical contact of the thing, the busy touching with its associated cozy, fleecy sensations, that satisfies most.

If you plan to introduce an animal to your own household, be sure there is someone at home to feed and care for it. AD patients usually cannot be counted on for consistency in this matter. Choose pets with soft coats, fluffy manes, and *very* pleasant dispositions—demented patients will unwittingly do outrageous things to animals.

Note that in some day care centers, volunteers make arrangements with the local SPCA to bring dogs and cats to the center so that the patients can be entertained and the animals exercised. If it is not possible to keep a pet in your lodgings full time, you might consider working out a visiting arrangement with a local pound or a pet-owning friend—working neighbors who must keep their pet locked up all day are often extremely receptive to such arrangements. Also worth looking into are "visiting pet" programs offered by local veterinary associations. These organizations will sponsor and help schedule visits from pets to the homes of elderly persons. They usually maintain lists of local pet owners willing to participate in such programs.

Plants

Judith Rodin and E. J. Langer noted that after providing nursing home residents with plants to care for on a daily basis, these residents become "more active" and "happier" and show "significant improvement in alertness and increased social involvement in many different kinds of activities." The researchers concluded that providing such recreation, besides exercising a person's nurturant side, provides "opportunities for control over ongoing daily events," producing "higher health and activity patterns, mood and sociability."*

It is difficult, perhaps, to believe that such a small thing as plant care could have so powerful an effect on elderly persons. Yet people who have worked with the elderly ailing know full well that for an afflicted person, a little bit can be a lot. If your loved one has shown an inclination for plant care in the past, it is certainly worth providing a few easy-to-care-for houseplants (such as spider plants or wandering Jew), and seeing how it goes.

Children

Demented patients and preschoolers mix wonderfully. Children four years old and under have no preconceived notions of how people should behave, and elderly persons are usually delighted to have such wonderfully happy, nonjudgmental company. In some families, caregivers arrange regular visits between oldsters and neighborhood toddlers. You can make such events especially attractive for young participants by serving ice cream and cake, giving out small favors, and, if you care to go this far, decorating the room with streamers and balloons. This way a festive air prevails, and the children are more likely to ask for a repeat performance. Elderly and young alike can share such activities as coloring, drawing, playing with animals, singing, eating sweets, and making simple snacks together in the kitchen.

Toys

As mentioned in earlier chapters, there is some argument whether or not it is proper to give demented patients toys. On the one side it is argued that toys infantilize the already infantilized, lower already low self-images, and reduce persons to objects of ridicule. On the other side it is said that whatever makes a person happy is good. In all, most professionals feel that the toy question is a subjective matter, one that must ultimately be decided by the caregiver in charge. At best a compromise can be worked: In the early stages, when patients are still able to identify the concept of a toy and to associate it with childishness, it is probably politic to avoid their use. At a later date, when patients have lost their powers of discrimination and when any diverting, brightly

* "Plants in Patients' Rooms," *Journal of Social Psychology* 35:897–902 (1977).

colored object captures their attention, toys may be more appropriate.

Apropos of the toy question, an article by Gloria Francis and Anita Baly is worth citing.* The article, one of the few ever written on this subject, provides an evaluation of tests conducted by the authors on nursing home residents to determine their response to stuffed animals. After observing an experimental group and a control group for an eight-week period, the researchers concluded that stuffed animals constituted "another example of the introduction of very simple, inexpensive, and easily managed therapies for the infirm elderly. Apparently, having a new stimulus that is pleasurable to look at, touch, own, care for, and talk about makes a difference—a big difference—even when that something is a plush animal."

Which toys work best? Patients will usually let you know on this score. Snuggly toys like stuffed bears are popular with men and women alike, as Francis and Baly discovered, perhaps because all of us had similar bedtime friends in childhood. In general, elderly women respond more to dolls and to the type of feminine toys that girls played with sixty, seventy, eighty years earlier. Males generally prefer boats, cars, rubber balls, and the like. But there are no rules—trial and error will decide.

Arts and Crafts

Arts and crafts still remain among the most popular of pastimes for demented persons. Crafts offer excellent exercise for coordination and mental stimulation. They are creative and productive, with a wide range of projects to choose from, and, of course, they can be done anywhere, at home or at a center. Most important for caregivers, crafts tend to focus demented patients, involve them, and quiet them internally. The following recreations are all recommended:

• Potting and clay. Long after patients can no longer make actual pots or figures, they will continue to enjoy the feel of the wet clay.

• Cutting and pasting. Collect colorful picture magazines such as *National Geographic* and *Natural History*. You'll need paste, paper, and a pair of child's scissors, which patients then use to cut and paste to their hearts' content. Cutouts of all kinds are good: Patients can scissor out shapes from colored paper or make collages. Or they can draw pictures, cut them, and paste them into a scrapbook. Seasonal projects such as

* "Plush Animals: Do They Make a Difference?" *Geriatric Nursing*, May-June 1976, pp. 140–142.

drawing, cutting, and pasting pictures of birthday cakes, Halloween pumpkins, Thanksgiving turkeys, Christmas trees, and the like are all recommended.

• Drawing and painting. All you need here are some watercolors, colored pencils, or a box of crayons. Patients will be kept busy for hours with this equipment and will enjoy it when you praise their work.

• Folding. Collect a variety of fabrics with different textures: wool, velvet, leather, silk, and so on. Encourage patients to stroke these materials and fold them into squares. For reasons unknown, working with fabric has a particularly tranquilizing effect on many persons.

• Leaves and flowers. Collect dried leaves in the fall and winter, flowers in the spring and summer, twigs and assorted branches any time of year. Participants will enjoy fashioning arrangements of these items, pasting leaves on paper, drawing ink prints and tracings, and pressing flowers.

• Making presents. Elderly persons can be encouraged to make an arts and crafts project and to give it as a present to friends or family members. Taking this approach often supplies a motivation that is otherwise lacking. Drawings, watercolors, clay figures, tracings, collages, flower arrangements, and the like all make touching gifts.

Other Recreations

Bear in mind that the activities suggested in this chapter so far are just that, suggestions. They are designed to stimulate your own ideas and to provide examples of the types of pastimes that demented patients have found gratifying in the past. Here are a few more ideas to consider:

• Gardening. Green thumbs endure. Onetime gardeners will still enjoy watering, planting seedlings, mulching a garden, digging in the soil, picking flowers, potting plants, harvesting vegetables, weeding, and all associated lawn and garden work.

• Kitchen work. Mixing ingredients, shucking corn, shelling beans and peas, scrambling eggs, making ice, setting the table, and other simple kitchen procedures are usually within the capabilities of early to moderately handicapped patients.

• Bird watching. A feeder perch can be attached to the window of the patient's bedroom, or an inexpensive hanging bird feeder can be located nearby. The person can be prompted to fill the feeder with seed each morning (purchasable at most supermarkets) and observe the birds as they come and go during the seasons of the year.

- Housework. Patients can be helped to feel both useful and, even more important, normal by being put to work. Try assigning household chores such as dusting, sweeping, or waxing. Erstwhile handymen will often still be capable of performing simple fix-it chores around the house or such relatively uncomplicated labors as painting, sanding, washing the car, and cleaning the garage.

- Making a scrapbook. Persons will enjoy compiling a scrapbook filled with family photos or pictures of animals, sports stars, scenic locations, postcards, magazine pictures, newspaper clippings, cigar bands, or other collectibles. Some caregivers encourage family members to keep three or four such paste-in books going at once. Much pleasant time can be spent poring over old picture collections, cutting up magazines, or pasting scrapbooks.

- Looking at picture albums. Most patients derive enjoyment from leafing through old picture albums, even when they can no longer identify who's who or what's what. Providing a running commentary of names, dates, and places will help in this regard. Sometimes patients in the later stages of dementia will momentarily recognize a face or place. They will point to it, say the person's name, or smile. This can be a gratifying moment for everyone. Album perusal has the added bonus that it can be enjoyed by the entire family at once, children included. Albums and old family photo books come highly recommended.

Exercise for Demented Patients

Watch an AD patient go through a round of exercise at the hands of an involved caregiver and you will quickly realize that the benefits of exercise are as spiritual as they are physiological. As a general rule, all demented patients should be exercised once or, better, twice every day, if possible, seven days a week. Exercise will keep joints flexible, improve circulation and elimination, and burn off excess energy or, conversely, rouse a sluggish constitution. It will entertain, divert, and enliven. It helps.

What kind of exercise is best? It depends on current state of health and stamina level. For persons who are ambulatory and who retain reasonable amounts of movement in most major joints, a round of regular calisthenics is best. Ideally, sessions should run approximately fifteen to twenty minutes a day, morning and night, but many patients will not be able to maintain concentration for this long. Says Jeannette Richardson, registered nurse and senior training associate at Brookdale Center:

You must realize that although you plan a twenty-minute exercise program, the patient may soon lose interest in what she's doing. So what do you do now? Well, you go through five or ten minutes of your regular calisthenics, then you let the person spend the last five or ten minutes just moving around, waving her arms and legs, getting the activity. Persons like to just float around sometimes, like children do when they dance. It doesn't really matter if they actually perform formal exercises. What's most important is that they move briskly, breathe deeply, and get a certain amount of physical stretches and rotations of their joints.

Dancing

Jeannette Richardson believes that one of the best and most enjoyable forms of exercise for AD patients is free-form dancing. "Use ballet music," she says, or any kind of music that matches the person's taste and culture.

Up in Harlem when we're working with Alzheimer patients, we use jazz and Eubie Blake. With other persons we use swing, waltzes, ballet, or classical— let it be the kinds of tunes they've danced to before, so that their body will have the right kinds of associations with the music. Then I encourage persons to just move around the room and dance. Nothing too fast or overstimulating. Just sway and move to the music and have fun. Everyone does.

Calisthenics

A vigorous set of gentle calisthenics offers excellent lifts and stretches and can be practiced as long as the person's attention lasts. Make sure persons do not strain, overstretch, or push beyond a comfortable level of endurance. Most persons will enjoy exercising to music. Supervise all sessions for patients who are in questionable shape or whose balance is wobbly.* Excellent exercises for those in good health include the following:

- Bend over and touch toes. Repeat twice. Do this exercise only if the movement is comfortable.
- Stand straight. Stretch the left hand to the right foot (or as far down as is comfortable), then the right hand to the left foot. Repeat five times.

* Dementia patients who also suffer from back trouble, high blood pressure, or other chronic illness should be advised by a physician before beginning an exercise program. In many cases the physician will want to tailor the program to the patient's needs.

- Extend both arms above the head. Stretch the arms as high above the head as possible. Return them to the sides. Repeat this stretch three times.
- Shrug the shoulders five times. Rotate the shoulders in their sockets five times.
- Go up on tiptoes, down, up again, down. Repeat five times.
- Hold the arms out in front. Rotate the wrists five times.
- Rotate the head, once clockwise, once counterclockwise.
- Extend the arms straight out to the sides. Rotate arms in small circles for approximately thirty seconds. Extend the arms in front and repeat the same movement.
- Sitting in a chair, lift the right knee, rotate the foot at the ankle joint three times in each direction, and return it to the ground. Repeat with the left leg.
- Sitting in a chair, lift the left knee, then the right knee. Repeat ten times.
- Sit in a chair. Stand up. Sit down again. Do briskly five times in a row.
- Take ten deep, slow breaths.

Exercises for Persons in a Wheelchair

Similar rounds of exercises can be done by wheelchair-bound persons, minus, of course, the moving around. Many demented patients confined to a wheelchair are by this point considerably incapacitated and will often need careful prompting and supervision. Appropriate music can be played during the exercises, as for other patients. Note that the number of repetitions given with each exercise are suggestions; they can be increased or decreased according to the person's capacities. The following movements are all safe and tested:

- Rotate the head clockwise and counterclockwise. Extend the neck and head upward several times. Bend the head down toward the chest, then backward toward the spine. Repeat three times in each direction.
- Sitting in the chair, extend the arms over the head and stretch them as far upward as they will comfortably go. Return the arms to the sides. Repeat five times.
- Shrug and rotate the right shoulder several times. Repeat with the left shoulder.

- Sit up in a rigid posture, concentrating on straightening the back and stretching the spine. Then slump back into the chair. Straighten again. Repeat five times.
- Extend the arms straight in front. Rotate them in their sockets for ten to twenty seconds. Wiggle the fingers for several minutes, and open and close the hands. Patient and caregiver shake hands several times. Caregiver says, "How do you do?" with a big smile each time.
- Extend the arms straight in front. Rotate them at the wrists for ten to twenty seconds.
- (For patients with some leg movement) Sitting in the chair, lift the right knee. Rotate the foot at the ankle joint three times in each direction, and place the leg back on the leg rest. Repeat with the left leg.
- Sitting in the chair, lift the right leg as high as it will comfortably go, return it to the leg rest, and repeat. Do ten repetitions. Then do the same with the left leg.
- Take ten deep, slow breaths.

Exercise for the Bedbound

For persons confined to bed or forced to lie on their backs, the following stretches will work against atrophy of muscle tone and will put most of the major joints through their full range of motion. It is especially important that the bedbound be exercised or contractures (shortening of the ligaments and tendons) will result. These cramping spasms can be extremely painful and will sometimes eventually force patients into a permanent fetal position.

- Lying on the back, lift the left leg up as far as it will go, hold it for several seconds, then slowly return. Repeat for the right leg.
- Lying on the back, lift the left leg and rotate the foot at the ankle for several minutes. Repeat with the right leg.
- Lying on the back, lift the left leg, bend it at the knee, and bring it to the chest. Straighten the leg and slowly return. Repeat with the right leg.
- Lying on the back, stretch the arms out and up. Rotate the arms in the sockets, then the wrists. Continue until this movement becomes uncomfortable.
- Lying on the back, lift the head off the pillow, extend it upward a

comfortable distance, hold it for several moments, then return. With head on pillow, turn the head to the right, then to the left several times in a row.

- Lying on the back, lift the left leg, cross it over the body, and stretch it to the right as far as it will go. Maintain this stretched position for several moments, then return. Do the same in the opposite direction. (Use this exercise only if it is comfortable and does not interfere with back problems.)
- Take ten deep breaths.

A Few Tips About Exercise

1. Mimicry is an extremely important process as far as the handling of a demented person is concerned. If you stand in front of a person and perform an exercise, the person is likely to copy you. Stretch your arms over your head. The person will do the same. Touch your toes. The person will follow. Mimicry is often an excellent way to get the sick person to do what you want, especially when words and coaxing fail.

2. Make sure all stretching is done to its maximum potential. Try to exercise all parts of the body, especially the major joints.

3. Supervision may be necessary for persons who suffer from balance or vision problems. Keep an eye on such patients during the exercise period and stay close by. Be prepared to catch them if they become disoriented or if they take a tumble. Even better is to let balance- or vision-impaired persons exercise while holding on to the back of a chair or to a nearby railing.

4. Since AD persons are easily distracted, be sure that all exercises are simple and require as little thought as possible. Complex combinations are not only difficult to understand but can prove frustrating and embarrassing for persons who suffer from motor difficulties.

5. Cardiovascular and aerobic types of exercise are, as a rule, too taxing for the elderly demented. Deep breathing is better. Have patients close their eyes, place their hands on their hips, and take three or four deep breaths in a row. Rest, then take a few more. Encourage deep breathing throughout the day. If patients have a heart or lung ailment, check with a doctor before recommending any kind of cardiovascular stimulation.

6. Caregivers can make sure that bedbound persons who are demented to the point of total incomprehension receive proper exercise by moving their arms and legs for them and by putting their limbs through

their full range of motion movements at least once a day. Do as follows: Stretch the bedbound patient's left arm out from the side. Pull it gently, move it from side to side, and rotate it several times in its socket. Repeat with the right arm. Next, stretch and lift the left leg. Rotate it in the hip joint, move the leg up and down several times at the knee, and rotate the foot. Repeat on the right leg. Finally, rotate the wrists, fingers, and head. This brief set of exercises may seem undramatic, but for a bed-bound person it can make the difference between comfort and agony.

7. Incorporate exercise into daily activity. When putting on a shirt, have patients stretch their arms above their heads and hold this position for a moment. When putting on shoes, have them bend down and touch their toes in the process. When watching TV, encourage patients to rotate their hands and wiggle their fingers. Have patients do a few leg lifts when getting in and out of bed. Let elderly persons help around the house; let them get some stretching when they reach to put packages away or bend down to pick up something from the floor. Encourage ambulatory persons to sweep, dust, mop, tidy up, fold laundry, or rake leaves. And remember, brisk daily walks are still the best exercise for young and old alike.

8. Always know a person's physical limits, and never exceed them. If you have any questions in this regard, consult with your physician before beginning any exercise program.

Reminiscence

Although short-term memory diminishes considerably in the early to moderate stages of AD, older memory patterns tend to remain more intact. Indeed, as many caregivers have remarked, the farther back a memory goes, the more likely it is to endure in a demented person's brain. Patients may not remember that they took a bite of corn thirty seconds ago, but they will recall that in 1922 in Denver, Colorado, they saw their first motion picture show in a theater called the Palace. Couple this phenomenon with the fact that few activities have as calm-ing an effect on demented patients as speaking about pleasant episodes from the past, especially episodes from childhood and youth, and you have the makings of a successful home care therapy. Indeed, some doctors are coming to feel that reminiscence sessions and related in-terpersonal communicative techniques are an efficient—and safe—means of sedation.

Reminiscence (or "life review," as it was originally termed by Dr.

Robert Butler, who developed the technique in the early 1960s) is a system that encourages elderly persons to recall and in a sense reclaim their own past—to look back, remember, and say, in effect, this is who I am and this is what I did and this is what I leave behind and this is how I feel about it all. Reminiscence can be done anywhere, at any time. It requires only a willing speaker and an interested listener-questioner. Normally it is practiced by intact elderly persons in an attempt to reinforce their sense of identity and to deal with the stresses of growing old. For demented persons, however, life review can also have profound value, especially in the early stages, but only when goals are kept modest and proper allowances are made for the person's reduced capacities.

Practiced with great success at the Brookdale Center for some time, reminiscence builds self-esteem. It allows patients to bypass their years of recent loss and to recall a time when they were clear and full of vigor, when they had energy, skill, authority, love. Reminiscence is thus of particular value among AD patients for whom past memories are often the only vestiges of individuality that still remain available. As an extra benefit, moreover, the actual act of remembering seems to stimulate memory function and is believed to help a patient's mind remain active for longer periods of time.

The reminiscence technique is simple. When employed in a home setting, it needs no formal training on the part of the caregiver. In a nutshell, it involves asking the elderly person a series of probing, specific questions about his or her past, then listening to the answers with attention and sympathy. After each reply, the listener puts forth another question or leading statement. Any emotionally relevant material is grist for the mill. Even substantially demented patients come away from reminiscence sessions feeling valued, happy, listened to, and complete.

Try it. Persons well along in their dementia can surprise you with the amount of information they are able to recall. For some these memories are all that remain, and they will be glad to share them with you as best they can. The following techniques, based on methods taught in several of Brookdale's training manuals, will serve as useful guidelines for keeping reminiscence sessions focused and meaningful.

1. Ask questions that require more than a yes or no answer. Don't say, "Did you grow up on a farm when you were a child?" Ask instead, "What kind of place did you grow up in when you were young?"

2. Use frequent prompts and supporting sentences to help persons

put their thoughts and feelings into words. Expressions like "you must have been disappointed when. . ." or "I'll bet it felt good after you. . ." or "It must have been hard for you when. . ." will help consolidate the speaker's recollections.

3. Focus on past skills and achievements. "You sound like you were really a good outfielder in high school." "How did you make so much money in one year in such a small store?" "You must have needed a lot of driving skills to maneuver a bus in all that traffic."

4. Solicit opinions based on the speaker's past skills. "Just exactly how do you cook squid anyway?" "Would you still invest your money in bonds in today's market, or would you stay with securities?" "What kinds of skills do you need to be able to identify a real pearl from a fake?"

5. Allow the person to share knowledge and skills. Let the person be the teacher and the teller.

6. Let the patient do the talking. Don't interrupt. Be brief in your comments, and concentrate on playing the part of listener.

7. Pick up on nonverbal cues. If the person's eyes show that a memory is too painful, drop it and go on to another subject. If a person starts to twitch or fidget restlessly at the mention of specific matters, avoid them. But if it looks as if the speaker wants to say something and is having trouble getting it out, be encouraging: "You look like you want to say something more about the bankruptcy proceedings." "It must be hard to talk about your daughter's accident."

8. Legitimize a speaker's feelings of anger or grief. "A lot of people feel angry at their children for leaving them—you're not alone on that score." "It sounds as if you really miss your wife."

9. Focus on emotions. "How did you feel when that happened?" "That must have made you a happy man!" "Boy, that sounds like it was a confusing time for you!"

10. Reminiscence is a feeling and sensory activity as well as an intellectual one. An odor, a song, a photograph can trigger a spontaneous release of memories. Cover all the senses:

- *Sight:* Use a wedding picture or an old family album to evoke a memory; use a scar on the hand, a necklace, a pretty sunset.
- *Sound:* Familiar music brings back familiar memories. So does the sound of a musical instrument or the words of an old song. Encourage the person to sing.
- *Touch:* The smooth side of a felt hat, a leather glove, a shaving

brush, the surface of a block of wood, anything that has specific tactile associations will help the recollection process.
- *Taste:* Certain foods will bring back certain memories.
- *Smell:* Smells bring back memories too. The French writer Marcel Proust based one of his most famous literary passages on a moment in which the narrator experiences a flood of childhood memories simply by smelling a familiar pastry.

11. Make use of nostalgic events and landmarks. Birthdays, holidays, religious observances, and important historical occasions can all become a focus for remembering. Ask persons what they did on Easter or Passover when they were children. Or what the mood was in America the day the stock market crashed in 1929. Or how things were the day Lindbergh completed his transatlantic flight.

12. Make your questions appropriate to the speaker's level of dementia. For those in the very early stages, most of the techniques mentioned so far will be useful. For those in the middle stages, questions must be pared down. A bit of trial and error may be needed to determine each person's current ability to narrate and recollect.

13. Don't pressure patients to answer questions. Let the session go on until they are tired or until their attention flags. If certain questions do not elicit a response, drop them and try again another time.

14. Use props. Some caregivers suggest showing objects dating from the person's youth, such as toys, washboards, magazines, clocks, and footwarmers, and urging the person to talk about their memories of these items. Drawings and photographs can also be used.

15. Reminiscence can be practiced anywhere and at any time. After a family dinner is a good moment to get persons to open up. Or in the evening, by the fire. Or before retiring. Or on holidays, birthdays, and special celebrations. The important thing is that persons be made to feel that their memories are valued. The more this feeling prevails, the more open and available they will become.

16. Never be critical or confrontative. Let persons know you care about what they think and the life that they have led. The enthusiasm and energy you bring to your expressions and voice tone are as important as the questions you ask. Really listen. Reminiscence sessions can be as educational for caregivers as they are therapeutic for the speakers. "There is nothing I like more," Socrates declared in Plato's *Dialogues*, "than conversing with old persons; for I regard them as travelers who have gone a journey which I too may have to go."

Reducing Stress: More Techniques to Help Make Patients Feel Better

Stress of some variety will be present among almost all dementia patients, as you by now no doubt know, and the techniques proffered here are all designed to deal with this difficult response. A few additional techniques for helping to reduce anxiety as demented persons go about their daily life follow.

Music

Patients who enjoyed music before they were sick will probably respond well to it now. Don't underestimate the sedative power of gentle harmonies, especially as a means for helping agitated patients sleep. Try playing a piece of familiar, cheerful music to persons who are deeply depressed or have just had a violent tantrum. Many will respond. A caregiver named Joan keeps soothing music playing on her stereo all day and reports that her demented father is visibly calmed by it. "The moment I stop the music," she says, "he becomes jumpy again. He asks me to 'put the sound thing back on again.' He especially likes opera music and ballet. Sometimes I play tangos or Benny Goodman because he liked those too when he was young. Good music is a great soother—it works."

Television

Though not all patients are unanimous in their affection for the tube, many respond to it gladly, and a few find it a positive soporific. Even after the action and dialogue are no longer understood by the severely demented, the colorful images produce a tranquilizing effect. Again, this is not true for everyone, and for some the effect is the opposite. Bill's family, however, found that whenever Bill became agitated and started pacing his room, if they simply turned on the TV and left it blaring during the night, it produced a sedative effect, even if Bill wasn't watching it directly. Some persons also enjoy watching movies on a VCR, especially older films that feature stars of the past.

Storytelling

Long after persons lose the ability to read, they can still derive pleasure from listening to stories. Simple, familiar, easy-to-follow tales (including fairy tales) are well received, as are reminiscences about shared experiences. Both can have a wonderfully quieting and mood-enhancing effect on listeners. As with any story, if it is told well, with gestures and enthusiasm, the listener will derive increased enjoyment. Some caregivers purchase book and story tapes and play them during the day for ailing family members.

Alcohol

This can be tricky, and not every caregiver will wish to include a shot of bourbon or a dry martini in the repertoire of stress relievers. However, for demented persons who have normally relied on alcohol for calming their nerves in the past or who simply enjoy the calming effect a drink has on the soul at night, alcohol can prove a welcome blessing. Consider the alternatives: chemical sedatives, tranquilizers, antipsychotics, physical restraints. Which would *you* choose if given the choice?

Reality Orientation

It has been found that when demented persons become disoriented, simply reminding them who they are, where they are, and what is happening at the present moment can often return them to equilibrium. During any activity, patients should be told where they are going, why they are going there, and what will happen when they arrive; for example, "We're going to the dinner table now. You are hungry. It's time to eat. We will have dinner at the dinner table. Are you ready?"

When Ralph first visited a day care center, his reaction was panic. Nothing was familiar. He didn't recognize anyone in the room; he didn't know where he was or why he was there. Consequently, he forgot who *he* was.

The volunteers acted quickly. One came over to him, put her hand on his shoulder, and said softly:

Ralph Nelson. Hello, I'm Irma. I'm your friend here this morning. Remember, Ralph, you're at the day care center. Your wife, Irene, left you here. She'll be coming back to get you in a few hours, Ralph. Remember now? You're at the day care center. You'll be here a few hours, and I'll make sure you have a fine time while you're with us.

A similar orientation technique establishing name, place, time of day, and situation in a firm, loving manner can be used whenever demented persons lose their bearings. All information should be said several times, and directions must be repeated throughout the course of an event. Avoid complex sentence structures. Speak in short, grammatically simple phrases. "Good night, Mom. It's time for you to sleep now. I'm going to turn out the lights. It's time for sleep. Good night." The best form of reality orientation is integrated into ordinary daily speech, so that demented persons do not realize they are receiving special treatment.

Reality orientation is an easy and useful technique that can enhance communication between caregiver and family member and help caregivers feel they are interacting productively with elderly patients. Try it at home and observe the results. The fundamentals of reality orientation, in review, are as follows:

1. If persons are disoriented, remind them of their name, the place, the date, and the event that is taking place.

2. Speak in a calm, kindly, noncondescending tone. Use short, simple sentences.

3. Allow the person plenty of time to respond. A few minutes may elapse before the message sinks in. If the person loses concentration or seems not to understand what you are saying, give the instructions several times.

4. When persons do acknowledge your words, reward them with a positive reinforcement such as a pat, a hug, a compliment, or a word of encouragement.

5. Make it clear to patients that you assume they will listen to and understand your directions, that they will comply with what you say, and that you expect them to help themselves to the full extent of their ability. Encourage persons to help out in their own orienting process. When a person asks questions such as "Where am I going again?" or "Why are we here?" this may be a good sign—it means the person is still involved enough to care about time and place.

6. Encourage other family members to keep demented relatives aware of reality by matter-of-factly reminding them throughout the day of where they are, what time it is, and what is going on. Instruct family members to do this in a natural and unforced way, as if it is simply part of the general conversation.

Order and Routine

AD patients tend to key in to their surroundings with great intensity, and any disorder or confusion can prove upsetting. For example, things out of place in the person's bedroom may provoke dismay or fits of anger. An object not kept within its usual context will cause patients to forget its functional purpose; for example, a hairbrush found in the kitchen will be used as a mixing spoon, and a pillow left in the bathroom will be used as a towel. It is thus crucial to keep the immediate environment neat and categorically organized—the shoes go on the shoe shelf, the urinal goes under the bed, the Kleenex goes on the table—and it stays this way. The same is true of the patient's routine: breakfast at nine, followed by a bath, exercise, a nap, and so forth. In general, it has been observed that the more structured and predictable a demented person's home is kept the more content that person will be.

Fatigue Avoidance

For many AD sufferers, fatigue has an agitating effect rather than a quiescent one. Such persons should have their daily events carefully monitored and should be encouraged to take frequent naps during the day. Limit all visits from friends to one hour, and politely cut all social calls short at the first sign of fatigue. Schedule taxing events such as visits, baths, exercise, and walks for early in the day when the person still has energy. Let the afternoons and evenings be for relaxation.

Quiet

Loud radios, rock music, several people talking at the same time, traffic noises, loudspeakers, and hubbubs can be disorienting and may trigger agitation. Be sure patients are kept in low-noise environments, away from sudden clanging and banging. If youngsters are in the area, make sure they use their radios and stereos in a far part of the house or apartment.

Humor

Nothing will pull you through the hard times better than laughter. Little jokes and pleasantries between patient and caretaker help clear the air, and it is surprising how some patients, out of it much of the time, will suddenly pop out with a golden piece of humor. Lucy, who was well on in the development of her dementia, urinated in her bed one day as usual and was in the process of being changed by her sister. Lying there silently for some time, as was her habit, Lucy suddenly sat up in bed, winked at her sister, and said with a twinkle in her eye: "By Elmo, I can still pee-pee and poo-poo with the best of them, Linda!" The laugh Linda got from this remark kept her going all day long. There is humor in even the darkest of situations. Whenever you see it, pounce on it. It helps.

Touching

Rosemarie, a nurse who deals with demented patients on a day-to-day basis, considers touching to be a first-class therapeutic tool and she often makes a point of frequently patting, rubbing, and caressing her charges while she speaks with them. She shakes hands with patients in greeting in the morning and hugs them in farewell at night. She explains:

Some people don't like to be touched, but most do. A lot. The more the better. You can have your patients who are babblers or wanderers and then you come up to them, put your hand on their shoulders, and amazing! They calm down. They feel good. Just like that. It's therapy for them. I think it somehow reminds them, hey! I'm still alive, I'm still part of the human race, aren't I? So during the day I try to make contact with the person's hand, shake hands, and look them straight in the eye. Or I'll put my hands on their shoulder while I talk to them. Sometimes you can kiss patients who are open to it, and they'll want to kiss you back. The ones who are really out of it and who keep their eyes closed all the time will make pleased noises when you comb their hair or pat their shoulder. Touching is a kind, warm thing all of us can do for the old and sick.

7

Coping with Abnormal Behaviors

AD patients may indulge in a sizable number of abnormal and even pathological activities at different stages of their illness, but certain behaviors are especially characteristic of the disease, and these are discussed in this chapter in terms of both what they are and what you can do to control them.

One significant thing to note about the bizarre ways in which demented patients deport themselves, however, is that many seemingly irrational forms of conduct—screaming, paranoia, wandering—may actually be the only remaining means by which the patient can successfully communicate with the world. Like a newborn child whose single tool for seizing power over the environment is tears, the severely demented person, whose mentality may hover not far above that of a newborn, is reduced to primitive grimaces and horrifying screams simply to gain a modicum of control.

Keep in mind, then, that abnormal behavior among severely demented persons, like all human behavior, may be a form of code. This code can be cracked at times, but at others it remains unfathomable, sealed inside the tormented glances or the indifferent stares of the sufferers. In either case, your job as caregiver is to do the best you can and to leave it at that. At a certain point along the line you will probably come to the conclusion, as so many other caregivers for demented persons do, that your best posture in front of all this is that of the pragmatist: If you can help the person, you will; if not, you will accept the status quo, look after your own peace of mind, and get on with living.

Determining the Cause of Problem Behavior

At a certain stage in the development of dementia, patients will no longer be able to tell you what they want. Their pants may be soiled. They may be hungry. Their shoulder may hurt. But they are simply no longer capable of communicating these facts. So instead they scream or cry or wander about or curl up into a ball. As with an infant, it then becomes necessary to use a process of elimination to determine what is behind their behavior.

Generally speaking, problem behavior can almost always be traced to three situational areas, detailed in this section. When a patient is in obvious distress but cannot, or sometimes will not, tell you what is wrong, you can often resolve the dilemma by reviewing these categories and asking yourself which one best fits the circumstance. Then you apply the appropriate remedy.

1. *The Environment.* Is the patient's room too hot or too cold? Is there need for another blanket? Is too much light streaming in through the blinds? Or is it too dark for the patient's needs? Are people in the area talking too loud? Are there too many visitors in the room? Also, consider objects in the surroundings that may have an intimidating effect. Curtains flapping in the wind will sometimes be perceived as snakes or grasping hands. Designs on wallpaper become ferocious animals. Loud noises outside the window can cause delusional patients to think they are being attacked. In general, give the person's immediate environs the once over when a problem behavior begins. Try to see the environment through the patient's eyes. Try to feel the environment the way the person feels it.

2. *The Caregiver.* Are you doing something that bothers the person? Perhaps he or she needs your company. If your voice tone is shrill, the person will quickly know you're angry and may react in kind. If your body language broadcasts messages of irritation or boredom, the person will become irritated too—remember, mimicry is one of the most typical forms of adaptive behavior among the AD population.

3. *The Patient.* Is Mother hungry or thirsty? Does her position need to be shifted in the wheelchair? Is nature calling? If she is incontinent,

does she need to be changed? Is she upset because she cannot tie her shoe or get out of bed? Is she depressed? Angry? Exhausted? Also consider physical ailments. Does Mother suffer from a chronic disorder such as arthritis, constipation, migraines, or back trouble? Could any of these be causing her to behave in a strange or unruly manner? What about bedsores?

After reviewing these three basic problem areas, jot down the factors you think may be causing the problem, and approach the patient directly. Sometimes a yes or no approach will quickly cut to the truth: "Are you cold, Mother?" "Is the nurse's singing annoying you?" "Is your side hurting you again?"

Some nonverbal patients will still understand what you are saying and can shake their heads yes or no when questioned. Phrase such queries in a slow, low voice at a steady cadence: "Are you hot, Mom?" (patient nods no). "Are you cold?" (no). "Do you want something to drink?" (patient nods yes). Interestingly enough, patients often maintain their ability to read and to identify visual images long after their speech skills fail. This ability can be a valuable aid for caregivers in a number of circumstances.

For example, James is a retired taxidermist who is now in the late moderate stage of Alzheimer's disease. His two sons and one daughter take shifts watching over him every day in his small apartment. Since James can no longer speak, a trick all three children now use is to show their father a card with an important word displayed on it. One card says "DRINK." Another says "EAT." Another says "BATHROOM." Still another says "GET DRESSED." And so on. A second trick that the family uses is to make stick drawings of various activities and to hold them up one at a time for their father to see. One drawing shows a person taking a shower. A second shows someone sitting in the sun. A third depicts a man sleeping in bed. And so forth. Whenever James becomes especially angry or restless, the combination of these two techniques goes a long way toward communicating and satisfying his needs. (A collection of useful pictures for AD patients is presented in appendix 2.)

Recalcitrant patients can also be bribed into revealing problems. As bait you offer an item the person especially enjoys, such as a candy bar, a snack, a walk, or some music. Persons are informed that if they tell you what's wrong, they will get the reward; if not, they won't. This method may sound mean and arbitrary, but it is not, really, as the patient's happiness is the ultimate goal. The golden rule is, if it works, do it.

Abnormal Behaviors and How to Deal with Them

Catastrophic Reactions

A so-called catastrophic reaction is an emotionally violent response to a seemingly insignificant incident; for example, a patient forgets to zip her skirt and begins slapping herself violently when she discovers it. A person is asked a question, cannot remember the answer, and starts cursing vehemently at the questioner. Typical reactions include crying, angry outbursts, verbal abuse, frenzied restlessness, and in some cases actual physical violence. It is the last of these reactions that gives caregivers the most concern.

Some patients go through a highly aggressive stage, acting out their rage in physical terms. They may strike out at caregivers or anyone else in the vicinity; they bite, spit, punch, or pinch; they lash out suddenly with a fist or foot when someone does something displeasing.

Strong, healthy patients, especially men, can become dangerous during such encounters, and everything possible must be done to quickly calm them down. Such carryings-on may indeed be part of the patient's frustrated attempts to communicate, but your foremost concern at this time should not be to decipher their hidden wishes but to get out of the way! The following steps will help you gain control:

1. Protect yourself. Get out of the range of the person's fists and kicks. Then hold up a barrier. Pillows make ideal shields, though in a pinch you can use a wastebasket, a board, or a chair.

2. Do not reason, plead, or try to talk persons out of their crazed behavior while they are actively violent. Now is the time for self-protection. Manipulate yourself into a defensible position.

3. If possible, back the person into a corner with the pillow or shield. Even strong AD patients will usually become tractable the moment after the violence has erupted, and physical aggression often ceases after just a few minutes. Make sure the person is maneuvered into a secure spot away from all doors. You will certainly not want your loved one dashing out onto the street at this moment and carrying the battle to the neighbors.

4. Remain silent while you are maneuvering the person, and try to keep the immediate environment as calm as possible. Screaming or scolding will only heighten the agitation. If you must speak, do so in a low, colorless monotone. Try not to communicate your anxiety. Staying calm is the most important thing you can do now. AD patients are imitative. If you're calm, they will become calm too.

5. Once the person is backed into the corner and quieted down, you can begin the dialogue. Be calmly reassuring: "I'm right here. I'm not going anywhere. I'm going to stay with you so don't worry. You don't have to be upset anymore. I know you're feeling worried, but you don't have to now. It's all right, you can relax and take it easy. Compose yourself for a few minutes and then we'll go have a nice cup of coffee together and maybe a piece of cake." Even if patients cannot comprehend exactly what you're saying, they will recognize the gentle voice tones and will no longer perceive you as a threat.

What You Can Do to Prevent Violent Behavior. There are four important things to remember about violent behavior patterns:

1. They don't happen very often.
2. They are usually over quickly.
3. Once the initial angry energy is spent, patients are just as eager as caregivers to get the ugly scene over with and they will usually give up without a struggle.
4. The violent stage itself is a brief part of the patient's course of illness, usually coming early in the illness and passing within a few months—which means that if families can weather this very unpleasant brief interlude, they will soon find that the patient becomes far more passive and manageable.

Another thing to keep in mind about catastrophic reactions is that they rarely occur out of the blue. Flash points are reached only after a certain number of failures and frustrations have accrued in the patient's experience, and because they have evolved via this cumulative process, violent outbursts can usually be linked to identifiable frustration-laden experiences.

What kind of experiences are we talking about? They are different for each person, but you would be well advised to pay attention to the moments in the patient's day that are particularly rife with perplexity and agitation (such as bathing or attempting to perform a mental task like reading). This holds especially true if the patient already has a history of violent reactions to frustration. Particular daily events that often discombobulate patients and set them off include these:

- Difficulties in getting clothes on and off
- Inability to comprehend what is being said
- Recurring problems with manual dexterity, such as having trouble turning a faucet or dialing a phone

- Failure at tasks that were previously second nature, such as frying an egg or remembering how to put a record on the stereo
- Disturbing programs on TV
- The realization that something obvious and important has been forgotten
- Confusion in the environment: new sights, new sounds, new people
- Being forced to think of several things at once
- An unexpected break in the regular daily routine
- Discovered incontinence
- Being offered help to perform a task that could previously be done unaided
- Being surrounded by angry or irritable persons

Another means of keeping track of potentially explosive moments is to examine the variables that may cause reactions. Suspect everything—the person's diet, the ticking of a clock outside the room, pajamas that irritate the skin, shoelaces that are difficult to tie, spices in the food, whatever. You never know. Pick out two or three of the most likely possibilities, and change them. Remove all salt from the diet. Stop the clock from ticking. Change the nightclothes. Switch to loafers. See what happens. If these changes don't do the trick, go through the same routine with a different set of variables.

Helpful in this regard too is to determine the times of day when persons go into rages, then to observe if these times correlate with a particular disruptive behavior. For example, when Larry was in the fourth year of his illness, he started throwing regular tantrums. Noting that these outbursts took place around eleven in the morning, Larry's wife soon determined that the problem stemmed from something quite ordinary: desire for lunch. Larry, it seems, was becoming hungry at an uncharacteristically early hour in the late morning. Since he could not communicate his needs in words, he conveyed them in a more direct way, by kicking, pounding the arms of his wheelchair, and generally carrying on.

You will often find that a primary cause of violent behavior is frustration at being asked to do something beyond one's capabilities. Putting on a pair of socks is an easy matter for us, but not for persons with dementia. For them it can be an experience that highlights their already festering sense of futility and despair. Address this situation by breaking down all tasks into simple steps. When helping patients dress, for instance, don't put all the clothes out on the bed at once. Hand them over one piece at a time. Make sure all goals that are set are attainable and that patients are not given chores beyond their abilities. Simplify, simplify, simplify.

Here are some more techniques for quelling catastrophic reactions:

1. Distract violent persons. Bring an unexpected object into their view. Say something that captures their attention. Turn on the television. Put on a fast, happy record. Take them for a walk.

2. Try physical tenderness. Violent patients will often calm down if hugged, petted, and lovingly stroked. Rocking angered persons in a rocking chair often has a tranquilizing effect.

3. If you consider a patient to be temporarily unapproachable, send tenderness and love through your voice. Talk in soothing tones. Let your intonations express fondness and serenity. If a person likes music, try singing.

4. Keep all body language unthreatening. If persons think you are going to hit them or that you are poising for attack, this will agitate them more. Maintain a bland expression, don't fidget, keep your hands at your sides, and don't make sudden movements.

5. Sometimes the best way to deal with catastrophic reactions is simply to ignore them, especially if they seem based on a need for constant attention. Simply let patients scream at the top of their lungs for a while or let them berate you verbally as much as they like. If you allow such behavior to run its course without reacting, eventually the behavior will disappear on its own, simply because it is not achieving its goals.

6. Don't use restraints unless the person is consistently given to fits of violence. If restraints are clearly called for, subdue only the parts of the body that are capable of striking out. After restraining the patient, reduce contact until the aggressive behavior subsides. Restraint of a demented patient is a tricky matter and should be discussed with a health care professional before being employed.

7. If a patient become physically unmanageable and cannot be quieted down, leave the scene and get medical help. If possible, do not go to the police. Call a local hospital or ambulance corps and have an ambulance sent. An ambulance corps is better equipped to handle a violent sick elderly person than the local police and they will have far more experience at it. This way you will also spare yourself any legal embarrassments—such as having an hysterical patient taken down to the police station for booking!

Dealing with Delusions and Hallucinations

A *delusion* is a fixed idea that has no basis in reality but is stubbornly maintained, even when the delusional person is confronted with objective evidence to the contrary. Thinking you are Napoleon is a delusion. So is believing that your son is a KGB agent in disguise. Most paranoias are forms of delusions.

A *hallucination*, by contrast, is a false sensory perception. Veronica actually thinks she sees snakes in the curtains. She actually sees her long dead husband and converses with him.

An *illusion* is a kind of small, momentary misperception of reality. A person looks at a hedge and in the twilight imagines for a moment that it is a prickly animal sneaking over the wall. The flashing headlights from a passing automobile cause a patient to declare that a fireball has flown through the living room. Illusions are usually experienced at night when shadows play tricks on the senses.

Both delusions and hallucinations characterize a relatively late stage in AD development, and not all patients suffer from them. Some do, however, and when they occur, the experience can be dismaying and disorienting for caregivers and patients alike.

Dealing with Delusions.   First, don't argue with delusional persons or attempt to talk them out of their folly. It doesn't work, and you'll soon be tied into knots. What's more, playing the voice of reality may cause you to be incorporated into the person's delusional schema, usually as a bad guy.

Never agree with a delusion either (or a hallucination, for that matter), and never play along with it. If a person tries to draw you into a phantom reality, stand your ground. Neither deny it nor affirm it. Instead, try to change the subject entirely and return the person's consciousness to the immediate environment. This can be done both verbally and with actions. The offer of food is a good distractor. So is taking the person for a walk, playing music, or making a mutual phone call to a friend. Speak of concrete things: what you will be having for dinner tonight, what the weather is like outside. Use diversion. Ask the person a question about a friend, about a favorite interest, about the health of a loved one. Solicit advice on a decision you must make. Give the person a massage.

In many instances delusions are an integral part of the person's ailment and, on the whole, are harmless. If this is the case, it is sometimes best to ignore them entirely. When Aunt Louise asks you if the president called from his office today, just say, "Not to my knowledge," and be done with it. If she tells you that her sons, both deceased, are coming to visit tomorrow, don't argue. There's certainly no sense trying to change delusional patients' minds or set them straight. At best we can simply get the persons' thoughts off their fantasies for a few minutes and keep them occupied. Caregiving is not remedial in this sense, nor can it be. Our goal is to make patients comfortable and reasonably happy; we cannot educate them or rehabilitate them. If we could we would but— alas!

Yet delusions are sometimes insidiously destructive, too, particularly when the gun is aimed at the caregiver. An elderly woman named Sarah in the later stages of her bout with AD turned against her loving husband of fifty-one years. Once an active member of several conservative political organizations, Sarah now projected her civic apprehensions onto her hapless husband, declaring him to be a "Leninist," a "fellow traveler," and a spy for "Lyndon Johnson's boys," whatever the latter meant. Whenever Sarah's husband came to visit, Sarah would ring for the nurses and announce that "the Benedict Arnold" had come again and would the nurses please report him to "the governor."

Needless to say, the pain these embarrassing encounters caused this man, himself almost a cripple now, was intense, and well it might have been. Watching such personality transmutations is one of the most difficult crosses the caregiver must bear in the name of the loved one. All relatives can do when it happens is to remember that it is the disease speaking, not the person, and that such pitiable fantasies are not the product of the familiar personality but of a mutilated brain. Caregiver support groups, discussed in Chapter 9, often advise caregivers on how to work through such encounters and how to put them in the proper perspective.

One way at least a modicum of positive value can be salvaged from a patient's delusions is to realize that these will-o'-the-wisps may offer cues concerning what the patient secretly wishes and fears. For example, demented women who constantly announce they are pregnant, a not uncommon delusion, may be reflecting ancient maternal needs and can be quieted down when allowed to visit more frequently with children. Persons who think their wheelchairs are automobiles may fantasize less if taken out for an occasional car ride.

One demented patient had a recurring delusion that her father, dead for decades, was about to arrive and give her a spanking because she had requested that the door to her room be left open. A perceptive caregiver realized that her sinister daydream was a covert plea to be taken out of the room more often. The patient's husband, the father figure of the fantasy, had made a point of keeping the door to the room tightly closed for fear that his wife would wander. In her intense state of paranoia, the woman was too frightened to ask that the door be opened and that she be allowed to go into other parts of the house, so she imagined her protection was a captivity.

Hallucinations. If a patient's mental faculties are extremely impaired and the person is experiencing frequent hallucinations, you can help by returning awareness to the concrete, physical world. Focus the person's attention on objects in the room: the colors of the wall, the wood on the floorboards, the bindings of books on the shelf. Try touching and stroking the person. Sometimes even light smacking and tapping on the shoulder, neck, and chest will snap the person back to reality.

Tender, supportive words can work wonders. Tell the riled patient you are here to help. Be direct and directive. Take charge. Tell the patient to sit up or stand up. Get the patient active and moving, or, if more appropriate, have the patient sit down in a chair and relax. Open the window for fresh air. Bring the patient into the bathroom and wash his or her face—water can have a strong grounding effect on a hallucinating person. Walk the patient around the room, assuring him or her that you are here and that the hallucination will not hurt. Stay calm and confident. When Rita's mother suffered from nighttime hallucinations, Rita would confront her fantasies directly:

> I'd say to my mother, "Oh, Mother, you must feel awful seeing these things." (She saw rats running up the side of her bed.) "Here, let me cover your eyes. Put your head under my arm till you stop seeing them." Then I'd pet her and stroke her and sing to her in Armenian (that's her native language) while she nestled in my arms. Sometimes this worked and the hallucinations would get less. Even if they didn't stop, they didn't seem to bother her as much when I was holding her.

In cases where hallucinatory conditions cannot be corrected by natural means, neuroleptic medications are often the method of choice. These drugs tend to work quite well for hallucinations, even in low doses.

Note, finally, that in some situations both delusions and hallucinations stem not from the actual dementia but from a physical disorder leading to delirium (delusions and hallucinations are considered to be delirium, not dementia). Drug toxicity, kidney infections, bladder infections, prolonged urine retention, dehydration, intense pain, chronic alcoholism, and many other physical stresses can trigger delusions and hallucinations. If you have suspicions along these lines, contact your physician for advice.

Paranoia

Closely related to delusions, paranoia is prevalent enough among demented persons to be considered in a category of its own. A seventy-nine-year-old woman demonstrated a classic paranoia by constantly accusing her two great-grandchildren of stealing her spectacles. She sometimes made this accusation while the glasses were resting on her nose. No matter, the notion that someone was out to steal from her had become an *idée fixe*, and no one could persuade her otherwise. Such is paranoia.

Dealing with Paranoia. In some cases paranoia will be a simple continuation of an already suspicious nature. In others it will be vaguely based on real-life concerns. The grandmother who was so worried over the theft of her eyeglasses was, in point of fact, becoming increasingly forgetful. Instead of perceiving her memory loss as an organic deficit, she projected the cause onto the outer world, making her great-grandchildren responsible for the mistakes she herself committed.

Blaming others for one's difficulties is common among AD patients, whose judgment and ego strength are both rapidly eroding. In truth, it is difficult for us to imagine how confused and disoriented demented persons feel inside, especially in the early stages of the disorder when they are forced to deal with the loss of faculties once taken for granted. How embarrassing it must be to forget your address, to be unable to figure out how to blow your nose, to continually lose your hat or comb or dentures. *Someone* must have taken those dentures. *Someone* must be responsible for misplacing the hat. A scapegoat is needed—this is surely an abiding human symptom in good health as well as bad—so someone in the patient's vicinity becomes the fall guy. Paranoia, in this sense, helps disoriented persons cope with and make sense of their environment. Their accusatory fantasies help them rationalize situations they could not otherwise understand.

Don't argue with paranoid patients or defend yourself if accused. Such reactions will only make persons distrust you more—challenging their opinion is further proof that you are against them. And don't tell the persons that they are "acting paranoid"; this will cause embarrassment and may even trigger a catastrophic response. Instead, deal with the problem on a purely logistic level. If eyeglasses are continually misplaced, keep a spare set on hand for when the originals are "stolen." Find out where the "stolen" object is usually left, and look there the minute it disappears.

If money is involved, as it often is, make sure paranoid persons keep their valuables in a safety box. If you are performing financial duties once handled by a sick patient, keep careful records of all transactions and produce them when questioned. Irma, when forced to become the check writer and bookkeeper of the house, got around her demented husband's money paranoia by cultivating a relationship with a friendly official at the bank. Whenever accusations about stealing money were hurled at her by her husband, she would call that nice Mr. X at the local branch office and put her husband on the phone. Mr. X would then assure her husband that all his accounts were in perfect order.

Here are some further steps that will help defuse paranoia:

1. Become the patient's confidant. Encourage the patient to tell you all about the details of his or her mistrust. Don't agree, but don't argue either. Bill yourself as a trusted listener, not one of "them" who are causing all the trouble.

2. If possible, keep the patient away from large groups of people. Paranoia tends to increase in crowds.

3. Empathize with a patient's paranoia. Say how hard it must be to think you are being watched, how painful it must feel to believe that so many people wish to hurt you. Some patients will know deep in their hearts that their fantasies are deviant and untrustworthy. Simply by sympathizing and letting the person vent, the paranoia can sometimes be softened.

4. Whenever you are about to participate in an activity with paranoid patients, explain to them beforehand what you intend to do. Never spring sudden surprises on such people. They may panic.

5. If a person confronts you directly with a suspicious accusation, brush it off lightly, give a brief explanation, and either change the subject or, if the matter revolves around something that has been "stolen," try to find the missing object.

6. Explain to all visitors beforehand that the patient is paranoid and that visitors may become a target of the patient's accusations. Friends

and associates are usually not prepared for such personality changes in the person, and they may react inappropriately if not forewarned.

7. Antipsychotic drugs and pharmacologic therapy may be called for when a person's suspiciousness reaches extreme proportions. Consult with your physician if the patient's paranoia becomes unmanageable—there are a number of drugs that can help.

Babbling and Repeating Actions

In the later stages of AD, patients may chatter nonsensically or repeat the same word or action many times in a row. Patients at respite centers can often be seen "sanding," moving their hands back and forth endlessly across a table. Marcia, a demented person, was obsessed with running her hands over her hair hour after hour. Ben would stand up and sit down hundreds of times in an afternoon. Liston pronounced nonsense syllables like "kakakakaka" or "brrrrrrrr" a thousand times in an hour.

Dealing with Repetition.   The cause of such troubled behavior is not well understood. In some cases, repetitious activity is harmless and not worth trying to correct. Sanders, strokers, rubbers, and preeners who quietly persevere are best left to their strange preoccupations. More disturbing, however, is verbal repetition. Sometimes caregivers can divert patients from this litany by clapping loudly, making a diverting noise, or in some cases telling the person to quiet down. One caregiver had luck keeping a patient busy by putting him to work doing specific activities such as coloring or stuffing envelopes every time he started chattering. But another caregiver was less fortunate. She tried to hush her noisy father by sitting in front of him, holding her finger to her lips, and emitting a long, insistent "shhhhhh." Her father, in turn, put his finger to his lips and repeated the same sound back. He then proceeded to say "shhhhhh" for the rest of the afternoon.

Whatever tricks you may come up with, chances are that in a few minutes the repetitious behavior will start up once again. Sometimes the only thing to be done is to leave the room and return later on when the behavior has ceased. Repetition, mercifully, does not usually develop until the late stages of Alzheimer's disease.

Restlessness and Wandering

Restlessness and its logical conclusion, wandering, are a major concern for everyone involved with demented persons, both because they can become so irritating and because they can be perilous, involving risk of injury, legal action, and even death. AD patients have inadvertently walked in front of trucks, started fires, driven cars into walls, and been arrested for masturbating in the middle of a city sidewalk. Clearly, it is better to keep the wandering patient safely at home, under lock and key and a watchful eye.

Why do demented patients wander? No doubt for several reasons, though if a single underlying psychological cause could be isolated, it would probably be linked with the search for an illusive security. For some persons the internal agitation level is so great that like a character in a Greek play driven by the Furies to wander forever, they are compelled by their very arms and legs constantly to keep moving. In other cases, patients are on an unending futile search, looking for some unfindable person, some unattainable place or thing from the past. A homebound patient named Ginger walked furiously up and down her hallway calling out "Mommy, Mommy!" all day and all night. Roger, a patient in a nursing home, was continually telling others that his wallet had been lost; he was several times found on the nursing home lawn, searching for this phantom object in the bushes. Other demented men and women simply seem to be aimlessly and endlessly drawn from one stimulus to another, agitatedly going to the wall, to the bookcase, to the desk, back to the wall again, for no other reason than sheer kinetic momentum, like pinballs. In each case the result is the same: a frenzied, perpetual compulsion to keep body and mind in constant motion.

Wandering and high agitation can occur at any time, but in many persons they become particularly prevalent in the evening hours. This nighttime phenomenon is known as "sundowning." Sundowning persons are docile during the day but become infused with a ferocious energy around eight or nine in the evening. They may suddenly leap out of bed, shed their clothes, and spend the rest of the night pacing the room, rattling the door, or even rolling over on the floor and jumping on the bed. Some patients shriek obscenities for hours or call out a single repeating phrase. Others pound on the walls or cry for hours on end. Rocking, clapping, doorknob rattling, and surface rubbing are all types of self-stimulation typically practiced by wanderers.

Why such frantic conduct only at night? No one is quite sure, and we can only hypothesize. For one thing, after the lights go out, the sensory stimulation of friendly voices and familiar sounds is reduced, and this silence can be a source of particular terror for AD patients. Feeling like prisoners alone in the dark, AD patients make noise simply to hear their own voices. Sometimes they are hungry or overtired. They may even be in pain and not be able to communicate this fact other than by agitated pacing. All the supports and human contact offered by a day's activities are removed now, and since demented persons live only in the present, with no sense that tomorrow is another day, nighttime wandering is often nothing more than the frantic search to reestablish the familiar.

Controlling wandering behavior.   Medications can be given to control wandering but they usually leave persons in a groggy condition; if the dose is not accurately monitored drugs can backfire, producing even greater agitation. Thus, if it is at all possible, try to control wandering behavior without recourse to medication for both your benefit and the patient's.

How? A number of drugless strategies have, in fact, been developed by trial and error through the years. Workers at Brookdale rely on several of these techniques, most of which attempt to lower a person's stress level, which in turn reduces the urge toward restlessness. Although none of these methods works all the time, some of them work some of the time, and that's a pretty good record as far as dementia goes.

1. Wandering can in certain cases be based on the need for more physical movement and increased dynamic social interactions. Patients should be kept busy with vigorous activities. Give them constructive jobs to do—housecleaning, arts and crafts, walks, baths. Going outdoors for a change of scene or taking a trip to the market or shopping center can be a tonic and may improve sleep quality too. For those who habitually indulge in agitated arm and hand movements, objects like rubber balls for squeezing, furry dolls for stroking, bean bags for shaking, and tops for twirling make excellent channels for restless energy.

2. Make sure wanderers' physical needs are taken care of. Agitation, especially among nonverbal patients, is sometimes due to hunger, soiled bedclothes, a cold room or a hot room, or even an actual ailment like a stomachache or back pain (arthritic and digestive problems tend to become worse at night for many persons). Before patients are put to bed, make sure they have been toileted and fed, appropriately medicated against chronic aches and pains, and comfortably bedded down.

3. Keep the environment free from disturbing sights and sounds. Noises in the hall can make persons think they are under siege. A carelessly discarded pair of pants hanging on the side of the bed can become the stuff of illusions and hallucinations.

4. Make sure patients know they are not alone and that other family

members are nearby. One of the primal terrors of the demented patient is abandonment.

5. Don't let patients become overtired. Fatigue will produce restlessness as quickly as lack of exercise. A happy medium between rest and stimulation should be maintained.

6. Sometimes simply using the powers of suggestion on patients can help them get their nighttime bearings and hence reduce their urge to wander. At bedtime, for example, the caregiving wife of an elderly stockbroker sits her husband on the side of the bed, rubs his shoulders for a few minutes, and caresses him lovingly. After the man is relaxed, his wife tells him that it is now evening. It is dark. It is time to go to sleep. Everyone in the house is going to sleep, and so is he. She tells him that he will sleep well and that others in the house are nearby. He is not alone. She repeats the messages several times in a row.

Though her husband seems only vaguely aware of what is being said during this routine, his agitation has lessened considerably since they began these sessions. Again, as in so many cases, though a person's conscious mind may not take in what is said, something down deep understands, especially when the message is repeated many times by a person who cares.

7. An agitated person's behavior may be rich in nonverbal clues that reveal the causes behind the agitation. It is thus a good idea to see if a person's wandering activities can somehow be connected to previous inclinations or to a person's past professional life. Sally, a helper at a Brookdale respite center, reports the case of an ex-businessman who was brought to the center by his daughter every day. Until lunchtime the man was a model patient and went happily along with the program. But immediately after eating he became wildly restless and constantly tried to leave the center through any exit he could find.

Finally, it was learned from his daughter that in the later years of this man's life, after he had become the boss of his own small company, he got into the habit of leaving his office after lunch every day and taking an hour's nap at home. On awakening he would then drive back to the office and work until seven-thirty at night. With this information in mind the volunteers at the center set up a cot for the man in the hallway, and each day after lunch they would let him lie down and snooze. Sure enough, an hour later he would pop up refreshed and rejoin the group happily until his daughter came to pick him up in the late afternoon.

Another woman at the same respite center would, like the man, remain inconspicuous during the mornings but turn wildly restless as the day progressed. She would walk up and down the two main rooms of the center rummaging through the wastebaskets, searching for scraps of paper, which, once found, she stuffed into her dress, tore up, and sometimes even ate. Eventually it was learned that the woman had been a secretary to an executive in a bottling factory for many years, which meant that her "paper chase" was perhaps somehow related to her past profession. Workers at the center started setting the woman up with secretarial supplies—envelopes, notepads, a stapler, pencils—and from then on she entertained herself happily with these materials, her compulsion to pick through the cans now greatly diminished.

8. An article in *Geriatric Nursing* puts forth a method for handling wandering patients which is called "agenda behavior."* The authors begin with the example of an elderly woman who has been recently hospitalized at a nursing home. During the evening meal the woman tries to leave the building, telling the nurses that she must go home and fix supper for her children. The nurses inform her that her children are fully grown. The woman responds by striking out at them, and the nurses in turn return her to the chair and apply restraints. The nurse then telephones the woman's physician, who prescribes a tranquilizer.

Must caregivers always orient persons to their setting, forcibly returning them to reality? ask the authors. Must they give the patient medication and apply restraints?

The authors suggest that when the woman headed off to feed her children, she was demonstrating a need to feel connected with people and to be of service. This was her true "agenda." By ignoring this hidden urge, the hospital staff aggravated the problem and precipitated combative behavior.

As an alternative the authors suggest that the nurses should have avoided arguing and instead should have supported the woman's emotional needs and even reinforced them. The nurses might have said something like, "I see, so you want to make dinner for your children? You must be a good cook. I'll bet you take fine care of your family. Are you worried?" By having her feelings reflected to her in this way, the woman senses that she is being listened to and understood by caring persons. As a follow-up, the nurses then take the woman by the arm (making important physical contact) and, talking to her quietly, gently guide her back to her room. In this way the patient comes to feel safe and cared for, and medication becomes superfluous. With appropriate mod-

* Joanne Rader, Judy Doan, and Marilyn Schwab, "Agenda Behavior," *Geriatric Nursing,* July–August 1985.

ifications, this technique can be used at home by family caregivers to thwart a loved one's wandering behavior.

The authors break their agenda method down into the following steps:

- Identify the patient's "agenda"—the emotions that motivate the wandering or agitated activity.
- When talking to the person, repeat specific words that relate to the person's agenda. In the example, the nurse uses words like *children, cook*, and *food*.
- Repeat the person's agenda. "So, you want to go home to cook dinner for your children?" "Oh, are you worried that your children won't get dinner tonight?"
- If the person does not respond immediately and continues to walk away, walk with the person and continue speaking, repeating the same messages several times and reidentifying the emotional themes.
- Provide orienting information to a patient only if it calms the patient or if the patient requests it. Otherwise, don't talk about the present situation or the fact that the person is walking restlessly about.
- At various intervals in the conversation, try to discourage the person's wandering by saying, "Let's go this way for a while." Then guide the person to his or her chair or room.
- Always speak to the person from a frontal position, being sure to make steady eye contact.
- If possible, touch the person lightly on the arm or shoulder while talking.
- Observe the patient's body language and nonverbal communication. Try to determine what this language is saying.

9. Sometimes a person may wander out of sheer boredom, releasing listless tensions through motor activities. This is especially common among persons confined to a room or kept secluded in a separate part of the home. In such cases the patient needs greater contact with others and more recreational activities.

10. If the patient is a frequent wanderer and actively attempts to leave the house, electronic devices can be installed to curtail these peregrinations. Some families place a closed-circuit TV monitor on the ceiling of the person's room. Others position alarms on certain doors of the house that, when activated, signal that the person is heading out of the house. Still

other families use one-way intercoms. Tamperproof locks and nonrattling, nonturnable door handles are available from most locksmiths.

11. All wandering patients should be made to wear some form of ID. The Medic-Alert Foundation International (1000 North Palm, Turlock, CA 95380) will, for a small fee, issue patients a Medic-Alert bracelet with their name and medical history on it, and this information will then go into a master computer, complete with the patient's private serial number. In the event that the person is found away from home, his or her name and address can be instantly traced by calling the number of the Medic-Alert Foundation given on the ID.

12. Experiment. A TV left on in the evening will keep some persons in their seats. Others use a radio or a chair placed next to a window, music piped in on the stereo, a snack before bedtime, tryptophan pills, chamomile tea—anything that works. Before you do anything, however, consider this: Though all the literature on AD bewails wandering behavior, do you as caretaker actually find it to be so bad? For some caregivers this activity is not a problem; it simply does not bother them or anyone else in the household. Patients, meanwhile, seem to find a deep and abiding satisfaction in constantly moving about. Sometimes it makes them happy and even euphoric. So what is wrong with it in these cases? Nothing.

You may even wish to help structure a person's wandering behavior. Find an area in the house or apartment free of obstructions and arrange a pathway between the furnishings to facilitate the person's pacing. Some caregivers have even painted footprints on the floor, which patients reportedly follow step by step with the greatest care and attention. Wandering is a strange and pathetic recreation, it is true. But if it harms no one, if the patient seems to need it, and if you don't mind when it occurs, why not let it be? It will then become one less problem you will have to think about for the day.

Self-mutilation

Demented patients often turn their confused energy against themselves. They may pick at their mouths till their lips turn to a grizzly pulp. They may hit their heads against a wall or pull out their hair. Scab picking and skin rubbing are common. So are nail and finger biting. One patient sucked her thumb so fiercely that several layers of skin peeled off before she could be restrained.

Controlling Self-mutilation.   Although it may seem that the patient is trying to self-destruct, self-mutilating behavior, it is theorized, stems less from self-hate than from stress run amok. Keep a close eye on the person and observe the style of self-harm indulged in. Sometimes simply keeping the person's hands busy will do the trick. Let persons draw, fold material, or stack coins. Increase their daily exercise, and make sure they get out of the house at frequent intervals to burn off residual energy. The idea is both to reduce stress and to keep the person busy.

Place all sharp or toxic objects out of the person's reach. Some caregivers try covering the mutilated areas with a bandage or gauze, though patients may simply switch their self-destructive attentions to different parts of the body. It is better first to attend to reducing the person's anxiety level. Many of the suggestions given above for reducing stress apply here as well.

Hiding and Hoarding Objects

Hiding and hoarding are not motivated by maliciousness as much as by fear and absentmindedness. Persons will use an object, shove it in an out-of-the-way place, and quickly forget it. A month later someone in the family finds the object behind a bureau or in the patient's pocket and explodes, convinced that the patient has become a thief. In fact, the patient has simply forgotten.

In other instances, patients will "steal" objects from the house and squirrel them away in odd locales. In Janet's household, Janet's husband and sister noticed that small kitchen objects were disappearing with increasing regularity. All these objects had one thing in common, Janet's sister soon figured out: They were silver and shiny—forks, strainers, tea infusers, and the like. Janet was quizzed and replied, in all honesty, that she knew nothing about the disappearing kitchenware. But a few days later her sister came upon the missing objects in Janet's upstairs closet. The items had been stuffed into the pockets of winter garments hanging in storage. Janet had done it, of course, though she denied it to the end. This is a typical scenario in the house of a hoarder.

Controlling Hiding and Hoarding.   When patients hoard or hide their own possessions, such behavior often represents a pathetic attempt at psychic survival. Demented persons have already had so many things taken away from them—their memory, their intellect, their coordination, their social life. All that remains are tangible possessions, and these last things must be saved at all costs. Seen from this perspective, hoarding is an understandable and deeply sad affair. Have patience with it.

If your loved one starts to walk off with your personal belongings, take all valuables, money, jewelry, and the like and stash it in a pro-tected, out-of-the-way place. A safe or strong box is best. To a hoarder, a diamond ring and a rubber band can be of equal value, and both will get flushed down the toilet with equal dispatch. Lock all doors that lead to vulnerable areas of the house, and get in the habit of keeping impor-tant things in places where the patient does not ordinarily go. You will, in essence, have to "hoardproof" your house. The ultimate goal is to keep the patient out of temptation's way.

Most hoarders have favorite hiding places that they tend to use over and over again. Find out where these stash sites are, and as soon as an object vanishes, check them out. AD patients tend to be creatures of habit—chances are you will find your missing goods in the same old places each time they disappear.

Inappropriate Sexual Behavior

Professionals are split over the question of how common sexual mis-behavior is among demented persons. Some claim they see it frequently; others see it only on rare occasions. Generally, the consensus is that inappropriate sexual behavior is uncommon and that when it does occur, it is part of a larger overall reduction of ego inhibitions. Typical sexual disruptions include masturbation, undressing in public, and exposing the genitals.

Dealing with Inappropriate Sexual Behavior.   Demented patients are usually uninterested in sex per se. Though their behavior may in-volve nudity or self-exposure, this does not necessarily mean that these actions are motivated by sexual urges. Quite the contrary, in fact; expla-nations for what appears to be outrageously lewd shenanigans are often quite innocent: A woman removes her blouse because it is too tight. A man plays with himself in front of visitors because his crotch itches. He takes his pants down because he wants to go to the bathroom.

The first thing you must do is determine whether the behavior is sexual or if it simply happens to involve a private part of the anatomy. More often than not, the latter is true.

At times behavior modification may help. If you see that Grandma is about to remove her underpants or reach for her genitals, a key phrase—"Hands off!"—used over and over again sinks in and prevents slips. In some institutions, when an inappropriate sexual activity is about to oc-cur, nurses will remove persons from the public setting, bring them to their rooms, point to a sign on the wall that shows a large green circle, and allow the forbidden behavior to continue here where it can now be done in complete privacy. Many years of association with this green symbol (for "go") will jog the patients' memory and remind them that such actions are verboten in public but permissible in the room. Repeating this action each time the behavior starts up can help set limits.

Still another technique used to discourage exhibitionism is punishment and reward. When persons perform sexually inappropriate acts, caregivers warn that if they do not stop the activity immediately, one of their favorite treats will be taken away—potato chips, a stuffed animal, television, cigarettes, beer, walks in the garden, whatever. When a person complies with this demand, the threatened item is then given as a reward.

Dr. Virginia Barrett brings another point of view to the subject:

> In my observation, persons' so-called sexual drive continues in a way after they're sick, but now it is not so much sexual as it is sensual. I have found that people who have had a recently active sex life now enjoy a lot of touching and stroking and sensual contact, and if they don't get it, they'll take it or do it to themselves. The whole thing is not necessarily intercourse-tied. Patients at this stage just want to feel good. It's a touchy-feely kind of thing.
>
> I also see that there is a lot of misperception on this question among caregivers. Caregivers have to ask themselves what is actually sexual and what is in the eye of the beholder. Sometimes I've heard visitors say that a patient's reaching out for them is a sexual act. That's how they perceive it—they perceive touching as sexual. But in actual fact, it's not that the demented person is thinking "sex" as much as that he or she is reaching out to establish familiarity and intimacy. Whether it's a breast or a shoulder is irrelevant. I think a lot of abnormal sexual behavior could be kept under control better if caregivers gave the patients more touching and stroking. That's what I think in most cases they're really after at this point.

Note, finally, that in some cases outlandish sexual behavior can result not from dementia but from the effects of medication. This holds especially true when patients begin acting in a suggestive manner out of the blue, with no prior history of exhibitionism. When it happens this way, check to see if the person is on a new medication. If so, contact your physician, who may consider reducing the dose, giving the medication less frequently, or changing it entirely.

Driving

The combination of reduced physical coordination and diminished mental acuity can add up to some pretty harrowing shenanigans behind the car wheel. Persons will go through red lights and stop signs with impunity, drive fifteen miles per hour on the highway, run people off the road or run them down, Keystone Cops style, all in blissful unawareness. It is a disaster, and family members are the ones responsible, both morally and legally.

The problem is further compounded by the fact that demented persons often deny their driving deficits as glibly as they deny their dementia. A driver who nearly sideswipes a truck and comes within an inch of smashing into a tree, all in one trip to the grocery store, will nonetheless grandly proclaim that there is nothing wrong with his eyesight, that it was the other guy's fault; it was probably even the tree's fault.

What to do? Family caregivers who suggest to drivers that they stop operating the family vehicle instantly become bad guys. Such suggestions have been known to catapult persons into tantrums and stubborn patients may double their efforts to continue driving. What is needed is an outside voice of authority, one that is both official and unimpeachable.

Such a voice does exist: It belongs to the physician.

Here, however, the plot takes yet another twist. An unexpected and perhaps unwitting ally in this drama is your local department of motor vehicles, which, it turns out, has the power in many states to prevent severely disabled drivers from operating a motor vehicle. They will discharge this duty, however, only if the doctor in charge writes a letter verifying that the patient does indeed have dementia and that he or she is indeed unfit to drive a car. The motor vehicles department, in theory at any rate, then takes the bull by the horns and removes the patient's license. But there is a catch. In most instances the job never gets done. The license removal law does not work very well. No one, it seems, wants to deliver the fatal blow.

Yet there is still a good deal of potential clout left in this situation if you are willing to tell a few white lies. What you must do is this: First, have the doctor write the formal letter on his or her letterhead, being sure the envelope is addressed to the department of motor vehicles in bold letters. Next, show a copy of the letter to the family member in question. Display the evidence as if it is a fait accompli, as if merely by sending it off the person's license has been automatically revoked. Blame it on the doctor, of course; announce that the doctor feels it is better for the patient's safety this way and that from now on family member X or Y must do all the chauffeuring. If the person objects, offer to call the doctor for verification. Usually even the most stubborn cases will cave in at this point and do what is in everyone's best interest anyway—not drive.

It is sneaky, but it may save a life or two, including the patient's—or your own.

Tough Love

When faced with a barrage of disruptive and abnormal behaviors, caregivers often have to confront their own resentment and anger. The first impulse when a loved one starts carrying on obnoxiously may be to walk out of the room or even to deliver a hard right hook to the jaw. This is an understandable impulse, of course, and a human one. Yet in the face of such a difficult situation, caregivers must manage to bite their tongues, swallow a few times, and get on with the job.

At the same time, caregivers should not make the mistake of thinking they must be total Milquetoasts in front of nasty patients or that being stepped on is a mandatory part of the caregiving deal. It's not. Caregivers can and should take a stand, balancing their love for the person against their need to control the person and to survive.

When raising children with this philosophy in mind, it is called "tough love." With elderly persons, it is the same. Tough love means the following:

- Don't be afraid to be directive and controlling. Though persons may act surly, most of them want to be told what to do, and if they are not given directions, they will find their own kind of mischief to get into. Words such as *no* and *don't* should be very much a part of your daily vocabulary.

- Use discipline when necessary. Though punishment and scolding are not successful tools in dealing with AD patients, when patients get out of control, you must stand your ground. If persons are being destructive, tell them to "stop *right now!*" If persons are throwing food at the table, say that they will go without supper unless they behave. If they continue to misbehave, isolate them until they come around. They usually will.

- When you become so exasperated that you can't stand it anymore, don't play the martyr. Escape temporarily. Have someone stand in for you and take a walk, do some exercise, watch TV, go to a restaurant, just get away and allow yourself to cool down. You are not a saint, remember. You have the right to get angry and to protect your turf.

- When children end up taking care of their parents, it is a strange role reversal indeed, and one that's not always easy to get accustomed to. Here's a daughter telling her own father to eat his supper, to go make a

BM, to hush up. It is all very strange, and for many persons guilt-provoking as well. But don't let it be. You are performing an important duty by taking care of your ailing parent, and it is part of the ancient, natural order of things. What you are doing is noble and fine. If you are uncomfortable at it, so be it. But remember, what you are doing is honorable and right. If you slip now and then and get angry, forgive yourself. It is a tough job, one of the toughest around.

Solving Behavior Problems

The disruptive behaviors mentioned in this chapter can all be controlled to one degree or another by using the coping strategies presented so far. Yet no one can ever formularize these matters entirely, and the care and feeding of an Alzheimer's person is constantly subject to the unexpected.

One way to stay on top of changes as they come along is to system-atize your approach to problem solving and to objectivize these problems by means of specific systems. There are many blueprints for such sys-tems, of course, but most are based on the same three steps: assessment, action, outcome. Here is one version that can help you: (1) Focus on the various trouble spots as they come up each day, (2) analyze the difficul-ties, and (3) plan tactics for overcoming them.

Assessment

You will need to note down when the problem occurs, what its consequences are, and what happens before and after. Reviewing your assessment will then reveal the origins of the dilemma, and solutions will in many cases automatically suggest themselves. A typical chart for such record keeping:

Time	Problem	Caregiver's Response	Outcome
Morning			
Afternoon			
Evening			
Nighttime			

Let's suppose that the patient has a wandering problem. Observe the person's behavior at different times of the day. Note the times at which the situation is best and worst under the heading "Problem," using a scale of 1 to 10. Under "Caregiver's response" record what, if anything, you did about the problem. Under "Outcome," note how successful or unsuccessful your response proved to be.

After observing the problem for several weeks and keeping careful records, study the chart and look for overall trends. Does the troublesome behavior tend to occur at certain times of day? What happens before it occurs? What seems to lead up to it? Are other persons involved? Who? Which of your responses seems to get the best results? How does your way of dealing with the situation help or hinder things?

Action

Once you have assessed and analyzed these data, make whatever changes are necessary. If the patient becomes restless before lunch, perhaps lunch should be served earlier in the day. If the patient is most tractable in the morning and worst at night, perhaps fatigue is causing the misconduct. More naps may be needed.

Outcome

Continue to record events after you make your modifications. Study them carefully and see what effects these changes produce on the person's behavior. How much has it, in fact, helped by making lunch hour earlier? If it has had a positive effect, the change is counted a success. If not, then another tactic will be required. Try serving lunch even earlier.

The sequence for solving the problem, in other words, is (1) keep records, (2) identify problems from reading the records, (3) develop interventions specific to the problems, (4) evaluate the outcome objectively, and (5) continue to make adjustments and changes until the problem is under control. Work carefully with the charts, and be creative in your analysis. Look for long-term trends and unexpected causalities. Play with your variables and use your intuition. You can apply this method to practically any problem related to the care and keeping of a demented person.

PART III

METHODS
FOR CAREGIVER
SURVIVAL

8

Coping with Your Own
Emotional Needs

Every caregiver's burden in this world is unique. It can be understood by others only after walking in the caregiver's shoes for an hour or for a day.

And yet, the concerns of Alzheimer's caregiving are somehow different from those of other terminal ailments, and in certain ways they are a good deal more insidious.

This is true for several reasons. With other fatal sicknesses, there is a built-in time limit. Family members can be confident that their loved one will die in a year, say, or two, certainly three or four, and they can prepare themselves accordingly. AD, being endlessly degenerative but never ultimately fatal, sometimes drags on for twenty years before the sufferer is laid low, and then the *coup de grâce* is delivered by a different disease. In many terminal ailments, the stages of decline are predictable and gradual. But with AD, random cognitive setbacks arrive daily; victims are dealt a series of continual symptomatic wild cards; nothing can be counted on, nothing is sure; from one point of grieving to the next and the next, there is always some sort of forfeiture to contend with, some sort of irreversible loss.

Persons dying from cancer or other degenerative disorders, moreover, grow thin and visibly waste away. Here is living testimony to the horror of this disease, and friends need little imagination to appreciate how difficult it must be for the sick person's caregiver. Not so with dementia-related ailments, where during the first few years the patient suffers relatively little physical degeneration and where sympathy and support from friends is equivalently scarce.

What's more, persons taking care of a sufferer of dementia are almost invariably heir to a very definable, very troubling collection of thoughts and feelings that are part and parcel of the ailment's development, feelings such as anger, helplessness, and the urge to run; guilt, disgust, and boredom; or hysteria, emotional fatigue, and despair.

The list is long, agonizing, and very typical—universal, even—and thus in this chapter you as caregiver will quickly discover that you are not alone, even when you experience the most outrageous and out-of-control reactions. You will see here and in the chapter that follows that there is help, and there are practical measures that can be taken to ease psychological burdens, and that these supports are no farther away than your car or your telephone.

Mourning the Living

Freud once remarked that the most difficult work people can do in life is to mourn for the dead. For the AD caregiver this notion takes a particularly ironic twist, as caregivers are forced to grieve for a person *who is not yet dead*.

This means that caregivers must not only live with the knowledge that their loved one will never get better but also must know in advance that the person will die by increments, on a day-to-day basis, and that they are destined to progress relentlessly from one point of grief to the next: Just as caregivers accustom themselves to one loss, a worse one comes along.

Also, caregivers must grieve for what is never going to happen as well as for what has already occurred. "I have to come to terms with the fact," an elderly woman said at a caregivers' support group meeting, "that George and I are not going to go to movies again, not once more. We're not going to go to Nassau together anymore in February like we always did. We're not going to share the pleasure of dinner at the Beaux Arts Restaurant anymore. It's over. I have to face this fact every day of my life. Over, over, over!"

Loss after loss. Eventually patients become dead before they are dead. Hear a caregiver named Leon on this subject:

I am in deep mourning, just as if I had my wife's coffin in the other room. I sit here and once the help goes home at seven o'clock all I need to do is turn my wife once and give her a drink of water before I go to bed. That's all. Between seven and nine o'clock I'm in my living room and a dead body is in the other room. Nothing. I'm sitting here with a corpse that's still breathing. This is not life. This is not death. What is it?

And yet, with such a terrible reality before one, there is also a splendid mercy. Each loss is, as it were, equivalent to a minideath. After enough minideaths have been mourned, the whole person is mourned as well, for in the act of grieving there is a cumulative effect. Says Rea Kahn, a skilled support group coordinator for the New York City chapter of the Alzheimer's Disease and Related Disorders Association:

> What we finally find is that for many people, when the patient dies, the caregivers have already done their grief work. The actual act is done. Especially when persons have worked in a group and talked through their feelings. As each deficit occurs, as the patient loses the ability to count or to socialize or to tie his shoelaces, this loss is noted and appropriately mourned. The outside world doesn't notice each of these minilosses, but the caregiver does. And each time the caregiver mourns, she learns to let go a little too. When the patient finally dies, she's well on her way to freedom from her attachments to this person. Because she's already done most of her sorrowing before that person has died.

For some people it is useful at a certain stage of mourning to program themselves into thinking that the patient is no longer here. Says Sylvia, daughter of an AD patient:

> This is not my father. He looks like my father, but I keep telling myself he's not. My father was a man of honor and love. This is just what's left over where my father used to sit. It's just a body occupying my father's former place. He's gone somewhere else now.

Take it a day at a time. Mark each loss as it occurs, and don't try to sweep it under the rug: It's here to stay. Recognize that even though the body in the wheelchair appears healthy enough, the mind inside it is declining, and with it the personality. This is reality. This is how it is.

Now is the time to grieve, to cry, and to begin severing the many emotional strings that, Gulliver-like, keep you tied to your former companion. As something in the patient dies each day, something in you will die too, until the death process is complete in both of you. What is important at this period is to realize that you are in a pattern of mourning and that this pattern has a beginning, a middle, and an end. No matter how endless it feels right now, it will not be forever. That's important.

Acceptance will help. In fact, acceptance is the key. Every day caregivers come face to face with the trauma and melancholy that deprivation evokes. They live with these feelings, dream with them, flail out against them, plead with them, repress them, flee from them, disguise them, distort them. They go through every conceivable emotional loop-the-loop imaginable to convince themselves that things can be different, that this is somehow not really happening. And when they are quite finished, they look up, and there is the demented person standing there, just as before, staring blankly ahead with the same impassive face.

Day after day of this, week after week, whatever the time span, and eventually caregivers begin to slow down inside, the angry energy of their denial and rebuttal spent.

At this point something relaxes and lets go. Instead of frantic avoidance, a kind of inner quiet dawns. In whatever fashion, via whatever route, the caregiver has begun to accept.

Talk to others about your feelings of loss and grief. Discuss the matter with friends, with fellow caregivers in support groups, with professionals, with anyone who is sympathetic or who has undergone a similar experience (you'll be surprised to discover how many people have). Their advice and recollections can help. Mourning for the living is an hour-by-hour, inch-by-inch process. Caregivers are well advised to practice it now if they wish to let go later.

Dealing with Role Changes

When Charley developed AD, he could no longer handle the affairs at the stationery business he had owned for fifty years. His wife, Rosa, had to take care of all the bill paying, the telephone ordering, the invoice programming, and the inventory sorting that Charley had been doing regularly since he was a young man.

When Charlotte developed dementia, her husband, Lou, took over her daily care. He learned to cook and to clean the house. He bathed his wife and did her soiled laundry and took her for walks. Voluntarily he gave up his job at the bank and moved into a nurturing homemaker's position.

Role changes. They come swiftly and decisively for the families of demented persons, and sometimes they throw everyone for a loop. How are they to be dealt with?

Dr. Virginia Barrett explains:

The real problem with role changes is not that the man suddenly has to do the housework or the woman has to fix the leaky roof. The real problem is that the expectations which exist between husband and wife are suddenly altered. Longtime spouses, you see, have usually honed their relating systems down to a finely tuned science. I do this job, you do that; I cook, you rake, I drive the kids, you drive to work: that's what marriage is all about. Things are set and established, and there's a lifetime of negotiating behind these patterns.

Then one day along comes Alzheimer's disease or some other dementia, and lo and behold, the husband can no longer walk the dog at night or carry out the garbage. The wife must take over these jobs, and chances are she'll get disoriented and angry at such new and, to her eyes, intimidating demands. It's not that she can't do it. Usually she can. Usually she copes. It's that the whole thing contradicts a lifetime of habit and expectation, and that can be very threatening.

According to Dr. Barrett, there are two ways of dealing with the anxieties that arise from role changes. First, start by pinpointing the task-oriented problems that are bothering caregivers and deal with them on a practical, fix-it level. Amy, for example, took over all financial duties when her husband got AD, and she was feeling very much under the gun about it all. Her therapist started by suggesting that she go to the bank right away, introduce herself to her husband's former contacts, tell them her dilemma, and have the bank personnel set up a financial arrangement that corresponded to her needs.

Amy and her therapist next went systematically down the list of remaining problems: How will the garbage be taken out? Who will answer the telephone when I'm out at my bridge club? How will the dinner get made on Thursday nights? Together they addressed each trouble spot from a purely logistic perspective and figured out ways of coping with each.

After these nitty-gritty problems were confronted, and after methods for negotiating them were devised, the therapist took things a step further. Moving into the psychological arena, she tried to help Amy realize that the real source of her anxiety was not paying bills, mowing lawns, or doing "men's work." It stemmed instead from the fact that her status quo had been disrupted and her systems had been turned upside down. This was the reason for the deeper upset and the source of her other anxieties as well. "You start by dealing with the circumstantial problems," says Dr. Barrett. "Then you work back to the problems behind the problems—fear, resentment, the panic of being out of control. That way you cover the boards."

Dealing with Anger

"*I feel like killing him!*" you catch yourself thinking. You are not the first to have this thought. The daily care of a demented patient is fertile ground indeed for resentment and anger. Anger at what? At the fact that the patient takes up all your time and energy. Anger because your social life is in a shambles and your body aches. Anger because your friends have stopped calling you. Anger at the patient for deserting you, for the fact that he won't be there when you'll need him. Anger because nobody understands. Anger because you hurt. Anger, anger, anger—which breeds guilt, guilt, guilt. It is a terrible cycle, and a predictable one.

Rare are the caregivers who have never entertained notions of using the patient as a punching bag or of simply walking out the door forever. Anger is a totally natural reaction considering the situation: You feel trapped; you feel frustrated; you are bored, hopeless, misused, and harassed. What human being would *not* react with such feelings?

The point is that when anger and resentment become an issue, caregivers' most important job is to forgive themselves and to realize that this response is unavoidable and universal.

Of course, once you've realized that you're behaving in a normal, predictable way and that most other caregivers are in the same boat, the anger and resentment still remain. When the patient refuses to take his bath for the hundredth time or when he reaches over yet again and helps himself to all the food on your plate, patience snaps. You begin having those punching bag fantasies again.

What to do? Listen to Rea Kahn, ADRDA support group leader:

> When I hear of people getting so angry they want to hit the patient, I consider this a red flag; they need to get away from the situation. At this point I strongly recommend respite in some form, day care, help in the home, a vacation. A caregiver must learn to recognize the danger signs in herself and act accordingly. She should leave the room when her anger gets the best of her and not come back until she's cooled down. She should go for a walk, watch TV, just get away. This will release the feelings a bit and help her blow off steam.

Other steps a caregiver can take when feeling hostile toward a patient include these:

1. Identify the hot spots during the day when the angry explosions tend to occur; then concentrate on modifying the conditions that spark them. The best way of doing this is to maintain a daily log in which you

record the incidents that lead up to the troublesome transactions.

Start by keeping a separate sheet of paper for every day of the week. On each page, divide the day into discrete time units: early morning, midmorning, noontime, early to midafternoon, late afternoon, evening, and night. Leave an appropriate amount of space for each unit. Then, immediately after an outburst occurs and the memory of it is still fresh, jot down the details under the appropriate time slot. Note the following:

- What were you and the patient doing when the problem began?
- What started it? What was the reason for the conflict?
- In what room of the house did it take place?
- What happened before, during, and immediately after the event?
- What unusual circumstances, if any, attended the incident?
- How was the problem finally resolved?

After you've recorded this information for several weeks, study it carefully and search for trends.

For example, caregivers may notice that their outbursts occur in the midafternoon, around, say, one to three o'clock. This, it then turns out, happens to be a time when no one is at home but the caregiver and the patient.

What does this mean in remedial terms? Perhaps the caregiver is reacting to the isolation and needs more support. Perhaps the person feels abandoned. Perhaps what is needed is more backup, more buoying up.

Another indicator to look for on the chart are chains of events that lead to problem behaviors. Let's say you notice on the chart that a few minutes before a daily blowup occurs, the demented person starts the laborious process of undressing for a bath. A few moments into it he announces that he won't take his clothes off, that he wants to eat dinner instead. You plead, to no effect. So you stop, leave the room for a minute, then return and try again. This time the patient starts crying like a child.

Aha! *Here* is where the explosion takes place. Those all-too-familiar tears have put you over the edge; it is at this precise moment that you tend to lose control. By reconstructing these steps on paper, caregivers can identify the components that typically cause a problem.

Once the trouble spots have been located and the flash points identified, plan strategies for modification. What room are you usually in when the dressing incident takes place? The bathroom? OK, next time try undressing the patient in the bedroom; sometimes a simple change of scene will alter behavior patterns. What about companionship from one to three in the afternoon? The mere presence of family members in the household can alleviate stress on the caregiver, even if these family members are not actively involved in nursing care. If family members are not available, perhaps a home aide or companion could be hired for several hours each afternoon. Or how about arranging for friends to telephone or visit at this time each day?

Be inventive. Tackle each problem individually. Record it, analyze it for patterns, then figure out creative ways to improve it. If you alter enough of these small events in your life, in the long run they will add up to big changes.

2. Try to avoid situations that make you angry. If you know ahead of time that your spouse or your parent is ornery at bathtime, turn all bathing duties over to another person in the household. Learn to delegate authority when necessary.

3. Talk over your grievances with others. Don't hold them in. Don't suppress your complaints on the grounds that you are betraying your loved one. This may be an admirable loyalty, but it is also a misplaced one. Caretakers have rights too, and one of them is the right to ventilate.

4. If you feel angry, go ahead and let it out—but not at the demented person, who will not understand your anger and will probably be intimidated by it. Instead, leave the room and find a quiet, solitary place for letting go. Car interiors are excellent for this purpose; so are basements, bathrooms, and even closets. Pound on the bed, yell at the clock, pull at the towel, do whatever is necessary to relieve the pressure. Don't be embarrassed. Some caregivers who work with the Brookdale staff keep pillows handy for slapping and hitting when they feel irritated. Others have special rooms in the house where they escape to when things get hot and hostile.

5. Make use of a support group. Venting is what these groups are all about; here you will be heard and helped by others. It's a two-way street, which is one reason why groups come so highly recommended. You will find all the particulars in Chapter 9.

When Anger Turns into Violence

Like any emotional reaction, anger can go too far. It is one thing to entertain fantasies of beating up the patient; it is quite another to do it.

If you find that you cannot control your violence, if you are constantly entertaining homicidal or bizarrely aggressive fantasies toward the patient, or if you physically abuse the patient regularly, recognize these behaviors as danger signals. They say you need help—*now*. Consultations with a social worker or therapist, advice from ADRDA or other support organizations, increased respite, home aide support, more time away from the patient, even institutionalization of the patient may be necessary. Whatever you do, do it quickly—it only takes one slap or one kick to do the kind of damage that can never be undone.

The Silent Phone Syndrome

It's not exactly that friends desert you when the chips are down. The process is more subtle. First of all, friends feel embarrassed when they visit. The person they had so much fun with on the tennis court or over a drink is acting strangely indeed. Friends are not sure what to make of it when the patient reaches over and starts picking at their clothes or when he drools. They try to carry on a normal conversation, with all the social amenities. But too often it's a one-way street—after all, how does one make small talk with a person who will not speak?

Friends are equally tongue-tied with you, the caregiver. Everything they say seems to come out wrong—too glib, too clichéd, too trivial in light of the situation. They feel embarrassed and inadequate. And really, what *is* there to say in the face of such a catastrophe? Sure, they are good sports about it all. They smile understandingly and tell you how beautifully you're coping and ask if there's anything, anything at all, that they can do to help. But inside they are confused and—dare they think it?—repelled too, and a little frightened. They wonder if you would rather not be alone. You have so many things on your mind these days. Perhaps you'd prefer not to be bothered—after all, you have not called *them* in a while either. Perhaps it's better this way—at least until the patient improves a little. . . .

And so the friendship fades.

It is also extremely difficult for friends to understand just how tired you feel at the end of the day. Nursing a demented person is an all-consuming task, and by nine o'clock at night caregivers have all they can do to stay awake. Perhaps you are not particularly young yourself anymore, and anyway, you feel too defeated to socialize. You feel unattractive, rejected. Who would want to spend time with you in this state?

The phone goes dead on your end and on the other end. On the rare occasions when you do socialize, you chitchat about the latest movies and the state of the world—but clearly you do it out of a sense of social obligation. Inside you're feeling guilty about being away from the patient. Perhaps Mother is hot or hungry. Perhaps the aide didn't show up on time. Perhaps she's fallen down or she's choking on a piece of meat. Did you remember to tell the aide about her dentures when she eats? Your distant gaze and distracted conversation telegraph these worries to your friends. But not really understanding the situation, they take this aloofness as rejection. You've become pretty poor company, you tell yourself. And if the truth be known, you have. So you stay home even more.

In many ways, it simply has to be this way. Once you shoulder the obligation of nursing a demented person, many doors will close to you and will remain closed for the duration of your caregiving stint. The decision to remain at home with the sick person is your own. It's just the way it has to be right now.

Thus caregivers tend to become isolated. Some devote themselves so entirely to taking care of their homebound invalids that eventually they become homebound too. And that means trouble.

As a rule, therefore, caregivers almost invariably need to reach out more, to make an extra effort to call old friends, to summon up that last drop of energy and go to a movie or a ball game or a restaurant. Learning to reach out is a kind of skill unto itself, and one that has to be learned.

One especially helpful approach to this dilemma is to form a buddy system with other caregivers. These people *really* understand what you are going through now and these are the people who for the next few years will make you feel most comforted. Get out of the house. Attend support group meetings. Become part of the network. Members of support groups often make it part of their program to call one another several times a week and to get together for lunch, for drinks, for trips, for conversations. It's good. It helps.

Turning inward is fine in its place. But when carried to extremes, it can pave the way for depression and alienation. Caretakers who feel listless a good deal of the time or vaguely anxious or just plain dead inside should bear in mind that lack of human input over long periods of time can have serious psychological consequences.

So keep your lifelines out. The most important thing you can do now is to find the right balance between giving your time to the patient and taking the time off to give to yourself.

Dealing with Sexual Loss

Several classic sexual problems plague caregivers of demented persons, as workers at the Brookdale Center have observed through the years. Perhaps you or your loved one have experienced one or more of these problems. The first is increased sexual suspiciousness. Unreasonable accusations are suddenly hurled by the patient: The caregiver is having an affair with the doctor. The caregiver is sneaking out at night and running off to sell herself in prostitution. The caregiver is married to another person. Crazy—but common.

Paranoia, of course, needs little encouragement to make it focus on sexual matters, and when this happens, caregivers can be driven to the far ends of their patience. It is not just that these paranoid accusations are so outrageous or so far off base; it's that they so violently undermine the trust that has been built up between marriage partners for years. This is what hurts, what is so infuriating.

Paranoia is, as you know, an intractable pathology that cannot be argued or pleaded away. Some caregivers, however, have succeeded in role-playing it into submission. One man, for instance, dealt with his wife's accusations by first agreeing with them. "No dear, that mistress of mine is not in the closet," he would say. Then he would walk to the closet, open the door, show his wife that no one was crouched inside, and assure her that it was all right now, the mistress had left and would not be back. This naive bit of subterfuge tended to placate his wife's suspicions for several days at a time.

A second problem related to sexuality is the loss of inhibitions. A male patient tries to grab his nurse's breast. A female patient exposes her genitals to a group of people in a restaurant. A male patient suddenly unzips his fly and begins to masturbate while friends are visiting. It can get pretty rough.

Yet, as was pointed out in an earlier chapter, most so-called sexual misbehavior among demented persons is not sexual or even erotic. It is more a kind of reaching out for sensation, for attention, and for affection. The impulse is the same as that proclaimed on a certain message button popular during the 1960s: "If it feels good, do it." If masturbation feels good, then masturbate. If a breast looks warm and soft, grab it. Simple as that.

If caregivers are having problems along these lines, it can be helpful to increase the amount of physical contact given the demented person. Stroking, patting, hugging, rubbing—these loving gestures are appreciated by most AD persons and sometimes are desperately required. In many instances, sexual acting out is the patient's way of demonstrating fears and anxiety. The patient is often unable to articulate these needs. In fact, much so-called sexual behavior may actually be an oblique cry for help, and you will quickly know the degree to which this help is needed by the intensity of the patient's response when it is given.

Still another sex-related difficulty arises when the patient desires intercourse with the spouse-caregiver but the caregiver is unwilling. Certainly sex with a demented person can be an undesirable prospect, for several reasons. The patient may perform in a mechanical, emotionless way that is off-putting and even a little bit frightening. Or, on the contrary, the patient may approach the partner with grunts and wild shrieks. The variations are endless, but the reactions on the part of the caregiver are the same: repugnance and dismay.

The fact of the matter is that at a certain point in the progression of dementia, sex between a patient and a caregiver *is* no longer feasible, and a process of separation must take place. Health care professionals often suggest that couples in this situation start sleeping in separate beds or living in separate rooms. If a demented spouse's affections are persistent and unwanted, it may simply be necessary for the caregiver to say a shrill no and walk away. Perhaps there is no other method. Eventually the demented person's sex drive will diminish and ultimately disappear. Like so many other functions that define our humanness, sex will also become a casualty of this unyielding disease.

Sometimes, of course, sexual situations call for particularly delicate and even creative solutions. Some years ago before the advent of the VCR, a man who had previously been a model husband and who was now in the early stages of dementia began attending X-rated movies on a regular basis. His wife soon caught wind of this, and she subsequently discovered that watching these movies was one of the few ways in which her husband could calm down. The choice was hers. Too disoriented after the first year to find his way to the theaters on his own, yet needing this peculiar form of stimulation to ease his terror, his wife swallowed her pride and started taking her husband to the films herself. Friends were, of course, aghast when they heard about these visits, especially since the theaters were located in the sleaziest part of town. Yet in the judgment of this sensitive and refined woman, suffering through the indignity of porno films was a way of helping her beloved spouse cope with his terrible pain. Truly, there is heroism everywhere, even in the darkest of places.

How Not to Get a Martyr Complex

Bette is at home day and night in New York City taking care of her demented mother while her brothers, Neil and Warren, live in Philadelphia. Every four or five weeks Neil checks in by phone and demands a medical update from Bette. He then offers advice, usually with a critical edge to it, complains that Bette is doing this wrong, that wrong, kibitzes for a few minutes about how stupid the doctors are, and hangs up. That's it for now. Warren is more actively involved in the situation, to the extent that he visits his mother every month or so and tries to help Bette out financially. But he too is critical of the way Bette manages the home care, and he frequently tells her that he thinks it would be better if their mother came to live with his family in Philadelphia.

Bette, of course, feels put down and unappreciated. Yet, in the face of this lack of recognition and despite the taxing work, she refuses help. When her brothers insist that she make use of respite groups or in-home aides, she insists that she can't afford it—though she can. When her friends suggest that she let her brother Warren become more involved in the care process, she maintains that only she knows how to care for her mother. And when *anyone* suggests that Bette have her mother institutionalized, she blanches and changes the subject—institutionalization is the unmentionable in Bette's world, the ultimate taboo. Bette is a typical Alzheimer's caregiver martyr.

What is Bette doing wrong? Is it not a noble thing to dedicate one's life to a loved one? And does Bette not deserve to pursue this sacrifice if she so wishes? Yes and no.

Yes, because it *is* a noble thing to dedicate oneself to the constant care of a terminally ill person.

But no also, for several reasons.

First, because by refusing help, Bette, a woman in her early sixties, is literally endangering her own health. Not only does the physical strain of waiting on an eighty-year-old demented person take its daily toll, but the psychological mix of anxiety, worry, and guilt that Bette lives with on a daily basis is slowly sapping her forces. Perhaps Bette will become sick—perhaps very sick. *Then* what will happen to her mother?

In other words, the caregiver owes it to the patient to take breaks, to allow others to help out, to elicit professional advice, simply because without this outside assistance, the caregiver will collapse under the strain.

Of course, the martyr position, with its built-in halo effect, is a difficult one for friends and family to assail directly, and interested bystanders are often loath to suggest that a caregiver's reluctance to accept help may be due, in part, to guilt, pride, and self-punishment. Explains Dr. Judah Ronch, psychologist-gerontologist, consultant at Fishkill Health Related Center, and author of *Alzheimer's Disease: A Practical Guide for Those Who Help Others* (Cross & Continuum, 1989):

> When caregivers refuse help of any kind, I tell them that there's already enough pain in them now and that they're worthy of relief. I tell them that refusing to take the patient to a day care center for a few hours a day or refusing another relative's offer to help out with cooking chores or refusing to hire professional in-home help doesn't support anyone, least of all the patient. On the contrary, accepting help is the best thing a caregiver can do for the patient, simply because it assures that the caregiver will stay well and thus be able to help the patient that much more.
>
> Sometimes I suggest that caregivers start by accepting help on a time-limited basis. Just try it, I tell them; see how it fits and feels. After a while, I tell them, we can reevaluate the situation. If they really don't find extra help helpful—and they almost always do—I tell them we can take the appropriate steps to discontinue it. The important thing is that I start them thinking in this direction, in the direction of self-help. Caretakers, I believe, absolutely *must* learn to counterbalance what they put out with the supplies they take in. These supplies include professional help, family help, and time off. In this way caregivers retrieve some of the energy they've lost. Then they can recycle it back to the patient. That's how it works best.

Little Ways to Help Yourself a Lot

On one point all professionals and seasoned caregivers agree: When caring for an Alzheimer's person, you *must* give yourself enough rest and free time. The methods and means mentioned here will help.

1. *Take turns.* Let other friends and family members help while you go out to a movie, a restaurant, the home of a friend. Encourage others

to do their share. If possible, distribute caregiving chores evenly among all family members. Avoid loading them all onto one person's back. Write up a schedule and take turns: John comes to watch Mother on Thursdays from 10 A.M. to 5 P.M. Leslie takes the nights. Richard comes in on Fridays. John comes back on Saturday. And so on. If one person is performing most of the caregiving chores and if relatives wish to help but can't agree on what to do, each relative can write down the services he or she is most capable of contributing—driving, financial aid, phone support, companionship, nursing duties—and the caregiver can make the final choices.

2. *Get out of the house as much as you can*. Change your impressions for a few minutes every day. Stop staring at the same curtains, the same rugs, the same pale face. Get air and light and sun whenever you can; being cooped up too long is the stuff breakdowns are made of.

3. *Use the phone*. If you can't get out, use the push-button lifeline sitting by your bed. Call people: friends, family members, business associates, anyone whom you enjoy chatting with and who offers support.

4. *Keep busy with other interests*. If you like to read, if you have a hobby, if you keep a scrapbook, if you enjoy cooking, *keep doing these things*. They will help refresh your mind and heart. Don't give up the pastimes that keep you interested.

5. *Exercise*. And do it as much as possible. Check with your doctor concerning the best variety for your age; then make an exercise schedule and follow it religiously. Exercise will keep the juices flowing, remove toxins, make you feel a little more human and a little less waterlogged. This is an important one.

6. *Eat well*. Because they are so tired so much of the time and because it takes effort to cook, caregivers easily fall into the white-bread-and-candy-bar syndrome. This is a mistake. You owe it to the patient as well as yourself to stay properly nourished. Eat plenty of leafy greens, fresh fruits, vegetables, and fiber. Drink enough liquids—many caregivers who are home all day forget to drink enough fluids and become dehydrated. Don't overeat; be sparing of caffeine and sweets.

7. *Take quality time out*. Plan ahead, make sure that you are covered, then go! For a weekend in the mountains, a two-day stay at the home of relatives, a short vacation, a trip to the beach, whatever. Just go, do it, get away, change your impressions. You will be amazed to see how refreshed and renewed you will feel when you return.

8. *Seek out pleasant perks and strokes*. A good dinner, a favorite movie, a massage, a new dress—be good to yourself whenever you can.

You deserve it. It will help you feel better about yourself and about your situation.

9. *Maintain your sense of humor.* Although tensions build quickly during crisis situations, don't forget the dazzling power of laughter to make strong medicine more palpable. Remember, no situation is without its comical side or its light moments, and no one has ever gotten hurt by laughing. In the midst of confusion, suffering, and even horror, humor above all things can, with a well-timed wink or naughty giggle, remind people that the light is as real as the darkness and that the human spirit has the power to prevail over all the tragic things that may happen in this very difficult world.

Knowing When You Need Help

Is there an ultimate symptom a caregiver can look for that indicates the need for professional help? Yes, there is: If you feel you can no longer cope, it is time to get help.

This sounds simplistic, but it is a foolproof formula. The need for outside assistance is a highly subjective and personal matter that depends exclusively on a person's perceptions: So if you *think* you need help, you do. Period. When Albert became incontinent, his wife, Lotte, accepted this messy reality as a matter of course and faithfully kept to her nursing rounds as before. But when Gertrude's incontinence began, this straw broke her husband's back, and within a week Gertrude was placed in a nursing home. In other words, what puts one person over the edge the next will take in stride. But note: each of us *does* have a point at which we break. Whereas Lotte was unbothered by her husband's soiled pajamas, she might have given up had her husband become violent or started wandering.

Each caregiver has a particular personal threshold, and each must judge when this magic line is crossed. For one person it is a depression that will not lift. For another it is obsessive eating binges or uncontrolled feelings of violence focused with ominous persistence at the patient. Panic attacks are not uncommon among caregivers, and they come accompanied by actual physical symptoms: chest and stomach pains, sweating, nausea, dizziness. All these manifestations are cause for concern.

For still other persons the red flag pops up with bouts of prolonged hysteria, suicidal ideations, excessive fatigue, heavy drinking, dependence on sedative drugs, a habitual feeling of being out of control, or an overwhelming sense of loneliness and desolation. Whatever the breaking point, know that each of us has this point and that to go beyond it without asking for help is to endanger your deepest well-being and hence the well-being of the loved one as well.

But know also that once this point is reached, the caregiver has only to ask and assistances of many kinds will be forthcoming. This is the good news, and the important news. You can find out how and where to find this help in the next chapter.

9

Getting Help

There is an old saying: "Help is often nearest when it seems most far away." As caregivers pass through one dark night of the soul after another without guidance and without relief, they come to feel that no matter what they do, no matter how hard they work at caring for the patient, they are never quite up to the task.

And do you know what? They're right. They can't do it all. No one can. The fact is that at some point on the caretaking journey, every man and every woman will need a helping hand. All personnel who work in the field of dementia agree on this point. Doctors, psychologists, home care professionals, seasoned caregivers themselves all unanimously agree: No matter how skilled or willing, a person is incapable of shouldering the burden of dementia alone. Part of a healthy, sane approach to this job is a willingness to ask for help when help is needed.

If you live in a major American city, most of the resources listed in this chapter are probably available to you in one form or another. In sparsely populated areas, more effort may be necessary to gain access to these aids, though as awareness of AD increases in the United States, assistance programs are proliferating everywhere at a rapid pace. In the worst-case scenario, if you reside in a rural area far from a major urban center, you are still assured of finding at least one ADRDA (Alzheimer's Disease and Related Disorders Association) chapter within several hundred miles of your residence. Besides helping you with group support and information, this organization will refer you to local assistance sources that fit your specific needs. It's good to know that somewhere, someplace, the kind of help you need is available.

Here is a sampling of what you have to choose from.

Respite Aid

A respite is a rest, a brief vacation from caregiving duties provided for the caregiver by family and friends or by a professional health care service.

Respite takes two forms, professional and voluntary. The former includes a wide range of aids, the most common of which are listed here.

Professional Respite

- *Home health aides.* Home aides are health care workers trained in domestic nursing. They are ordinarily provided by home care agencies, which, in turn, are referred by health care professionals, support groups, or word of mouth.

Depending on the schedule you work out, home aides will come to your house for a certain number of hours a day and perform any of a dozen different tasks. They may oversee personal care chores such as bathing and toileting the sick person. They may move the person from bed to chair or expedite dressing and feeding. Aides will also perform basic nursing tasks such as taking vital signs, exercising the patient, and assisting with medication. In some instances they will be trained in domestic services as well: household chores (housecleaning, shopping), cooking, and even secretarial duties. Though costs for home aides vary from organization to organization and from location to location (urban services tend to be more expensive than rural), count on $8 to $10 per hour.

- *Companion services.* Also available from most health care organizations, companion services provide semiskilled aides to watch patients for a prearranged number of hours a week. Companions are capable of performing simple nursing services such as turning the patient in bed and helping the person move around the house. Costs for companion services run from $7 to $9 an hour.

- *Homemakers.* Likewise supplied by professional health care services, homemakers vacuum, make beds, dust, wax, mop, sweep, and generally keep a home tidy. They also help out with the more strenuous household duties: taking out the garbage, carrying groceries, opening the garage door. Usually hired on a once- or twice-a-week basis, typical costs run from $7 to $9 an hour.

• *Live-in aides*. When caregivers feel they need round-the-clock professional support, a live-in aide may be employed. Supplied by health care services, live-ins serve as general factotums and jacks-of-all-trades. They shop, answer the phone, and accompany the caregiver to the bank, hairdresser, doctor, wherever. They do light household cleaning, assist with menu planning, and help patients with grooming, bathing, dressing, and toileting activities. They also serve as companions and emotional leaning posts for caregivers on a day-to-day, hour-to-hour basis. Typical costs run from $100 to $150 a day. Some hospitals and home care agencies offer sliding scales.

• *Chauffeur services*. Chauffeurs will spare elderly caretakers the aggravation of driving or of having to deal with public transportation. Supplied by professional health care agencies, chauffeurs cost anywhere from $8 to $20 an hour, depending on the time of day and the company's rate schedule. The price can sometimes be negotiated down if caregivers plan to use the service on a regular basis.

• *Escort services*. Escorts take caregivers wherever they wish to go: a friend's house, the bank, the drugstore, the movies. They carry bags, open doors, push shopping carts, and provide general companionship. Costs run from $7 to $10 an hour.

• *Chore workers*. Similar to homemakers but with more muscle, chore workers tackle heavy-duty jobs: carrying packages, patching leaks, shoveling snow, raking leaves. Available through professional health care services, chore workers earn $9 to $12 an hour.

A Word on Home Health Care Agencies.   Most large home health care agencies provide all, or at least a majority, of the health care services just listed. But how can you tell the good agencies from the lemons? Though there are no foolproof methods, here is a list of the kinds of questions you should ask before making a decision:

• What specific services does the agency provide, and how much does each cost? How long has the agency been in business? Does it maintain several offices? Is it independent or part of a chain?

• How is the billing handled? Is the agency covered by insurance plans and Medicaid? Is it bonded? (This means that if one of their employees steals from your home, you receive reimbursement.) Does the agency maintain a sliding scale or part-pay program based on the client's income? Are there any hidden costs (such as transportation fees for aides)?

- Who provides general supervision and coordination of the in-home program? Does the agency offer a contract or service agreement stipulating its rates, services, specialists provided, hidden costs, hours of care, and the like? What type of emergency response system does the agency offer?

- Is the agency certified or accredited? If not, why? Is it for profit or nonprofit? Can it provide references from doctors or administrators at community organizations and hospitals? Ask for specific names of references, and call these people directly. What kind of training does the agency's in-home personnel have? Are references available for them?

- Does the agency provide home medical equipment? What types of equipment can it provide? What equipment is it *not* capable of providing? How does the billing work for equipment rental?

- During what hours of the day and night does the agency provide services—twenty-four hours a day, or just 8 A.M. to 8 P.M.? Are services available on weekends? On holidays? Are fees higher for services rendered during off hours? How much higher? Must you pay for a minimum number of hours even if you do not use them?

- What type of relationship does the agency maintain (if any) with your supervising physician? Has your physician ever worked with this agency? What does he or she know about them?

- Does the agency provide a complete (and free) home assessment before treatment begins? How thorough is the assessment? Will the agency reassess the home situation should the need arise? (Many agencies promise such assessments beforehand but deliver only halfheartedly. The interest and enthusiasm that home agencies display for your situation are critical.)

- Is there a personality match between the professional caregiver and the demented person? Mismatches are among the most common problems that crop up in home care. Are you happy having this person in your home every day? Does he or she fit in well? Is the person pleasant? Does the person do a good job? If not, you are certainly within your rights to ask for a different helper or to change agencies entirely.

Other Forms of Professional Respite. You may want to consider these alternatives:

- *Short-term institutionalization.* Some nursing homes accept patients on an overnight or weekend basis. The patient is checked in on, say, Friday night and leaves on Sunday. For caregivers this service provides a perfect compromise between the need to keep a patient at home and the need to rest and recuperate. Unfortunately, not all homes offer this service. Inquire locally or seek a referral from a health care professional.
- *Overnight in-home respite.* Some hospitals and nursing care agencies offer overnight services for the families of patients who must be away for days at a time. In such instances, professional aides come to the caregiver's home, sleep over, and attend to the patient's needs. Usually these aides come well screened (check on this, however), though their services may cost as much as $200 a day. Some hospitals and home care agencies will charge clients on a sliding scale.

Volunteer Respite

Volunteer respite is usually informal and inexpensive. It is available from the following groups:

- *Churches and synagogues* may offer volunteer companion services to senior citizens. Inquire locally.
- *Public schools* sometimes require students to log a certain number of public service hours working in the community. Helping the handicapped and the elderly sick is a frequent service offered. Inquire locally.
- *Community organizations* offer respite services for caretakers of senior citizens, though you may have to cut a bit of red tape to get recognized. A doctor, a social worker, or your local ADRDA chapter will refer you to the nearest agency. The following organizations can provide information on community-sponsored respite and home care in your area:

National Association for Home Care
519 C Street NE
Washington, DC 20002

National Home Caring Council
Division of the Foundation for Hospice and Home Care
519 C Street NE
Washington, DC 20002

- *Families* often work out schedules whereby each member contributes a certain number of hours a week to relieve the principal caregiver. If hours cannot be contributed personally, acceptable substitutes will often keep peace within the family. For instance, in one family, three sons live out of town and are not available to help their sister take care of their demented father. In order to compensate, the brothers chip in a certain amount of money each month to hire a home health aide, thus buying their sister fifteen hours of respite a week. Everyone is satisfied with this arrangement.

Adult Day Care Facilities

Though technically a form of respite aid, adult day care is so important a resource, designed as it is to provide recreation for demented persons *and* time off for caregivers, that it deserves a heading of its own. Privately run day care units can be expensive. The costs of centers operated by the state, university, or public service organizations (the Brookdale Center sponsors ten day care centers in the New York City area) are minimal, if not entirely free. Important to note about the difference between private and nonprofit is that with day care, what you pay for may not necessarily be what you get, as many nonprofit day care facilities are liberally endowed by foundations or universities and serve as training grounds for hardworking students and dedicated volunteers. Investigate the matter carefully before choosing. If possible pay a visit to the respite center first to observe things firsthand.

What does a typical day consist of at a day care center? Schedules vary from center to center, but generally the agenda runs something like this: The caregiver delivers the patient to the center early in the day, say, around 10 A.M. After being greeted by the workers (usually volunteers or trainees), patients are set to work at various activities. Depending on their level of physical impairment and mental competence, they may draw, play bingo, make art projects, listen to tapes and records, or simply socialize. Many centers emphasize group activities such as storytelling, singing, arts and crafts, listening to music, or exercising. At some centers patients dance to music or play catch with a ball. At others they participate in reminiscence sessions or go on short day trips. Still others provide therapeutically oriented recreations designed to improve memory, recall, and coordination.

At midday lunch is served, and later on, snacks. In the afternoon, usually around three or four o'clock (or early evening in a few cases), patients are picked up and returned home. Many patients attend day care activities every day.

The beauty of day care is, of course, that it offers caregivers a compromise between keeping demented persons at home and placing them in an institution. It also provides patients with a welcome change of scene and a chance to escape their own four walls, while for caregivers the precious free hours between breakfast and midafternoon can be weighed against gold.

There are several day care variations besides the one just outlined. At some centers, caregivers may, if they wish, remain on the premises with their patients all day and participate in the programs. Besides keeping contact with patients this way, caregivers get a chance to meet other caregivers, make friends, and socialize with men and women who are in the same boat as themselves.

Most urban areas and many rural communities now have adult elderly day care facilities of some kind—health care professionals or a support group such as ADRDA will provide you with names and referrals. Here is another organization that can furnish specific information:

National Institution on Adult Day Care
600 Maryland Avenue SW (West Wing 100)
Washington, DC 20024

Whatever form of respite you choose, just remember that the persons who staff these groups are pros and that even if your loved one suffers embarrassing problems such as incontinence, the workers here have seen it all and are well equipped to deal with almost anything.

Visiting Nurse Services

Depending on your needs and hourly requirements, visiting nurses will come to your home, help out with medical care, and oversee the patient's private needs. Though a round-the-clock nurse is usually not required until the last stages of dementia, caregivers who can afford the high costs of personal nursing will find that having a licensed professional on the premises at any stage is the next best thing to having your own in-house physician. A luxury, yes, but a blessed one.

Visiting nurse services provide two grades of nursing personnel: licensed practical nurses and registered nurses. It works like this:

Licensed Practical Nurses

A practical nurse is a graduate of an accredited vocational school or practical nursing program who has passed a state board of examination and is trained to perform a wide spectrum of skills under the auspices of a physician. Practical nurses will help develop a nursing care plan for the patient, administer medication, document the patient's medical progress, and provide high quality daily care. Typical costs per hour are $30 to $50.

Registered Nurses

A registered nurse is a graduate of an accredited college who has passed the state board examination and is licensed to practice with a physician and/or independently. Patient care responsibilities include performing medical treatments and administering medication as prescribed by a physician, documenting the patient's daily care, instructing family members in nursing techniques, maintaining a safe household environment, and continually assessing and updating the patient's home care plan. Typical costs per hour run from $40 to $60.

For more information on visiting nurses in your area, speak with your physician or a social worker, or get in touch with these organizations:

American Affiliation of Visiting Nurse Associations and Services
21 Maryland Plaza (Suite 300)
St. Louis, MO 63108

American Federation of Home Health Agencies
429 N Street SW (Suite S-605)
Washington, DC 20024

Professional Medical Services

In most cases, the process of hiring medical professionals will be initiated by a physician's recommendation, then instituted by a hospital or home health care agency. Health care professionals whose services are most likely to be required include the following:

Social Workers

Social workers will come to your home; assess the patient's (and caregiver's) logistic, social, recreational, and emotional needs; and make referrals or provide counseling. Social workers are especially useful when working directly with families. They will iron out internecine conflicts and help enhance intergroup communications. Social workers are referred by physicians, hospitals, home care organizations, or social work agencies. Their rates for in-home visits range from $40 to $60 an hour; some agencies bill according to a client's income and ability to pay.

Child Care Workers

In the event that children or teenagers live in a household where their parents' time is taken up caring for a demented relative, it may become necessary to hire child care workers for several hours a day. Child care workers are, in effect, trained baby-sitters. They escort children to school, pick them up in the afternoon, take them to the playground or to a friend's house, oversee homework activities, and keep the home running smoothly. If caregivers must be out of the house for several hours a day, child care workers will act as home coordinators or supervisors, making sure that all youngsters are fed and entertained. On the average, child care workers receive $9 to $12 an hour. They can be hired through baby-sitting agencies or home health care organizations.

Nutritionists

When unusual dietary needs arise, a nutritionist may sometimes be called in. One patient, for instance, may be protein-deficient yet unable to tolerate meat and dairy products. Another may be unable to eat but have a ravenous appetite. A third may be overeating but also showing signs of malnutrition. Such cases are best handled by a competent nutritionist. Nutritionists cost $40 to $60 an hour for in-home visits, a bit less if you consult them at their offices.

A different nutritional scenario occurs when caregivers are too poor to afford adequate meals or are incapable of getting to the grocery store to shop. In such cases, locally sponsored nutrition programs such as Meals on Wheels will bring free or low-cost lunch and dinner directly to the caregiver's home or apartment. Churches, schools, and synagogues often institute such programs, as do community and state-connected organizations. Inquire locally or at an ADRDA office.

Physical Therapists

Although the deficits that develop from dementia are ultimately irreversible, some professionals believe that regular physical therapy sessions help stabilize and even maintain a patient's eroding physical skills. Referrals are made by a physician or a hospital. Costs are around $50 per hour.

Speech Therapists

Speech therapists have reportedly had some success helping demented patients preserve failing language skills, as well as teaching caregivers methods for improving their communication skills. Speech therapists are referred by doctors or hospitals and are provided by hospitals or home care agencies. Costs are $50 to $70 an hour.

Occupational Therapists

Occupational therapists help patients cope with the small, round-the-house physical skills (such as turning a doorknob or getting in and out of a chair) that are necessary for maintaining normal day-to-day functioning. Costs are between $40 and $60 per hour.

Psychologists and Psychiatrists

In some cases the strain of caregiving becomes so great that caregivers require help from a practiced mental health professional. In Chapter 8 we dealt with situations in which therapy becomes necessary—depression, anxiety, alcohol and drug abuse, undue hostility toward the patient. As always, the decision to initiate therapy is a personal one, and no matter what friends or family members may think or say on the subject, if caregivers feel they need professional support, this feeling itself is adequate reason for getting it.

Referrals for mental health assistance can be made by your physician, support groups, or other caregivers. Positive word of mouth from satisfied clients is the best of all recommendations.

Professional Health Care Consultants

Yet another route caregivers can take if they are feeling especially under the gun is to use a professional consultancy service that specializes in helping families and caregivers of sick elderly persons find their way. What services do consultants provide? Though different agencies specialize in different support techniques, a well-trained consultant can serve in a number of vital areas. Marilyn Howard, director of educational services at the Brookdale Center and Codirector of COPE, a New York City–based geriatric consulting service (45 E. 89th Street, New York, New York), describes the process, using her nursing background as a cornerstone:

> A consulting service like the one we operate specializes in helping people feel they are not alone, that they have some control over the situation, that they are not the victims and dupes of an impossible system.
>
> For instance, one caregiver may need certain advice and referrals. So my partner and I will act as a clearinghouse. We'll tap into our own network of professionals and direct the clients to the resources which best fit their particular situation. Maybe this client requires the names of medical therapists, or inside information on a certain nursing home, or a good home aide, whatever. Maybe clients need advice on legal and financial issues like Medicaid, power of attorney, or third-party payments, in which case we'll refer them to one of the lawyers in our network who can advise them on how to spend their money and husband their resources. Each case is different.
>
> Sometimes, of course, the need is really acute. A family will be having terrific problems at home managing a patient, and they won't know which way to turn. They don't want to send Papa to a nursing home, but they can't cope with his wandering and violent behavior either. So they get in touch with a consultant service like ours, and first off we do a total evaluation of their situation. We come into the house, observe, talk to the family and patient, get the lay of the land, then give some preliminary advice, maybe tell them how to arrange the furniture in a safer way, how to control wandering within the setting of their home, how to improve communications between the home care aide and the patient, how to keep the lid on a patient's violent activities—anything can pop up. In other words, we analyze, make up a plan of care, then present the client with all the options. Once this is done, the consultant may then leave the scene and the client will use us again only on an as-needed basis. Or the client may require ongoing support and management. It varies from person to person.

Support Groups

In the opinion of many experts, a support group is perhaps the most valuable and dependable resource a harassed caregiver can turn to in time of turmoil and despair. Whereas friends may look away and family members fail to contribute their share, whereas associates may think they understand your dilemma but don't, whereas the world may minimize or even ignore the struggle you are engaged in every day, members of a support group are different. They have been there. They know from experience. They can help.

Support groups for caregivers of demented persons come in many shapes and forms, though undoubtedly the most popular of these is the ADRDA-sponsored support group. With chapters throughout the United States, ADRDA groups are run by highly trained specialists who know their stuff and who have usually been caregivers themselves. These groups meet every week or every other week, depending on the membership's needs, in hour-and-a-half sessions. Topics discussed range from methods for changing soiled bedsheets to finding a good home care agency to dealing with suicidal fantasies.

What advantages are to be gained by caregivers who attend support group meetings? There are many. The basic ones are therapy, education, and socialization.

Therapy

Though most support groups are not set up on actual psychotherapeutic lines, in many cases deep emotional and psychological issues are touched on as a matter of course during sessions. Members may use their meeting time as a chance to vent, to let emotions out. Or they may simply listen, ask questions, solicit advice. What they need is what they will get.

The leaders of most ADRDA groups, meanwhile, are trained in dealing with psychological issues, and though leaders ordinarily do not delve into members' psyches, they will often help members define psychological issues as they come up and hence gain greater insight. Says ADRDA support group leader Rea Kahn:

> I never allow any kind of personal attack in my groups, and I never try to rip away a person's defenses. The people who come to this group have made a contract to join a *support* group, and that's what we try to provide—support. Meetings here are therefore different from regular therapy in this sense, but they are like therapy in the sense that contact with other persons in the same boat as oneself can ultimately help members come to terms with the reality of their situation. It can help them become more accepting, and gain a better picture of their own strengths and limitations.

Education

Caregivers are the best of all resources for gaining practical information. How do you bathe a patient? Someone in the support group will know. Incontinence? Stress management? How do you get through the sundowning syndrome? What do you do when your demented spouse kicks you? How can you handle a patient who curses in public? What's the best nursing home in the city? Where can I rent a wheelchair?

Whatever your question, someone in the group will have an answer, a fact, a bit of advice, and you also will contribute your share. It's a give-and-take kind of exchange, and everyone profits.

Socialization

Since persons in support groups are, as it were, members of the same exclusive club and participants in the same ongoing drama, it is within the natural scheme of things that many will also become friends outside the meeting place. Indeed, for some persons, group members become their sole source of help during hard times, and the group becomes the constructive center of a life that is otherwise entirely negatively focused.

Support groups work. They really help. They put things in perspective and provide real succor. Yes, it is difficult for some caregivers to rouse themselves, to make that difficult phone call, to ask a stranger for help. But this is an effort that will be well rewarded; sometimes it's an effort that saves a life. Do it. Try it. Once caregivers start going to support groups, most find it difficult to imagine how they ever lived without one.

ADRDA

Beyond doubt the most prominent national organization now serving demented patients and their caregivers in this country is the Alzheimer's Disease and Related Disorders Association. Established in the late 1970s under the auspices of the famous gerontologist Robert Butler, ADRDA maintains chapters in almost every state of the Union and works tirelessly to help increase public awareness of the problems indigenous to dementia.

To squeeze all the extraordinary things this organization does into a few paragraphs would be impossible, and here we can only touch on its most significant activities, especially those that are directly helpful for caregivers. Be aware, however, that whenever you need help and advice on Alzheimer's-related matters, ADRDA should be the first place to which you turn.

Education

ADRDA works on many levels to educate the public concerning AD. Each year a large number of dementia-related materials are published under ADRDA's auspices—topic-specific articles, a quarterly newsletter, self-help pamphlets and brochures for caregivers—all of which can be ordered directly from their offices. ADRDA also offers videos on dementia-related subjects plus films, audio tapes, written reports, magazines, and pertinent books, all lent free of charge from their office library. Recently, a group of professionals affiliated with ADRDA has prepared a full-length book on AD titled *Understanding Alzheimer's Disease,** which is highly recommended for patients and caregivers alike. Other educational activities include a speaker resource bureau, public relations campaigns, fund-raising activities, lectures, seminars, and much more.

Services for Families, Caregivers, and Patients

Support groups are perhaps the most visible of all ADRDA services, but the organization offers several other important forms of assistance that concerned persons should know about. One of these is a twenty-four-hour-a-day free-access help line staffed by trained volunteers (all of whom were once caregivers) that provides advice and information on just about any topic relating to dementia. To find the help line in your area, look up ADRDA in the phone book, or get in touch with their main office:

Alzheimer's Disease and Related Disorders Association, Inc.
70 Lake Street (Suite 600)
Chicago, IL 60601
(800-621-0379; in Illinois, 800-572-6037)

Another no-fee support is ADRDA's medical referral service. At most ADRDA offices, a sizable data bank is kept, listing local physicians, specialists, hospitals, home care agencies, and useful resources. Employees at the ADRDA offices will make this information available on request and will refer caregivers to physicians for first or second opinions, to medical specialists, to diagnostic clinics, to nursing and home care facilities, to therapeutic organizations and counselors, and to local help groups and organizations.

* Miriam K. Aronson, ed., *Understanding Alzheimer's Disease* (New York: Scribner's, 1988).

Research

Since ADRDA was founded, it has earmarked more than $7 million for dementia research, according to John A. Jager, New York ADRDA chapter executive director. "And that's a lot," says Jager, "for an organization that started out with seven little local chapters less than a decade ago. This increasing amount of research money is, I believe, a cofunction of the education and advocacy policy that ADRDA is trying to spread."

Advocacy

Alzheimer's disease is a relative newcomer to public consciousness, which means that donations are far less forthcoming than they are for other killer diseases. As Dr. Ken Davis, prominent researcher in the field of dementia at Mount Sinai Hospital in New York City, explains:

> Although Alzheimer's disease funding has moved up in the past few years from a pittance to fifty or sixty million dollars a year, this amount pales in comparison to the money allotted for other diseases. There is currently a *billion* dollars being spent on AIDS research. Not that AIDS isn't a terrible health hazard; but AD is far more terrible, ranking as the fourth-largest leading contributor to death in this country. Per patient, Alzheimer's remains a grossly underfunded condition. If we don't want the next generation to suffer from the same plague as this generation of patients, it requires a commitment of the national will to help out.

ADRDA is doing its part. As different legislation comes up in Congress, ADRDA works hard to keep its constituency aware of the issues at stake. Through a planned policy of advocacy, the organization informs members concerning changes in national funding for health care and new bills up for passage—bills, say, that sponsor increased statewide day care units or more generous social security benefits. ADRDA also takes political positions with other health organizations and tries to rouse local chapters to back public policy issues that really count. Wherever controversial politicomedical issues are being debated, ADRDA will be there, championing the good guys.

Thus: If you are in charge of a demented person and want to connect with the best clearinghouse for dementia resources currently available in the United States, investigate ADRDA and contemplate membership. Whatever you are looking for, whatever you need, chances are excellent that someone in the ADRDA organization will have it for you.

Institutionalizing the Demented Person

At what point does it become necessary to place a demented person in a nursing home? The answer to this agonizing question is as varied as the personalities of the people who must make the decisions. For Glen the moment arrived when his wife became hopelessly incontinent. For Gale the line was crossed when her father lost his ability to speak and no longer responded to her affections. For Arnie institutionalization was necessary when his wife became both blind and violent. For Shelly it was a purely financial decision: He could no longer afford to pay for full-time nursing care at home. Many persons, many motives.

Is there a single underlying incentive behind these decisions to institutionalize? Dr. Virginia Barrett has studied the question of institutionalization for many years and believes that behind the standard reasons given for placement, such as incontinence or wandering, lurks a hidden emotional catalyst that is deeper and more difficult to quantify: the patient's ongoing ingratitude and indifference toward the caregiver.

> When a doctor is trying to find a bed at a nursing home, that doctor must come up with some hard-core reasons to prove that the bed is needed and that the patient is too deteriorated to live at home. Thus when the doctor finds out that the patient is indeed incontinent, he or she will write this down on the person's papers as the grounds for applying, and this gets plenty of points when the application is reviewed at the institution. Often, however, as our interviews and studies have shown, the *real* reason the caregivers are having this patient sent to a nursing home is not because the caregivers are tired of changing the patient's soiled undergarments or because they can't put up with his petulance. It's because they feel so *unvalued* for their efforts, so unloved and ignored and unacknowledged by the nonresponsive Alzheimer's sufferer. *This* is what evidence frequently shows to be the underlying motivating factor behind the decision to place.

Whatever the ultimate provocation for bringing a patient to an institution, there is little doubt that such a decision will be among the most difficult caregivers will ever be forced to make. Though no one can promise to relieve the oppressiveness of such a difficult task, approaching it from a systematic and informed perspective is always the best—and ultimately the least painful—strategy. Let us review briefly what caregivers must know about the process of institutionalizing a demented loved one or family member.

Where to Start

Once you have made the decision to place, the next question is, What kind of facility will I put the person in? There are several to choose from, including these:

Foster Care.   Offered in some but not all states, foster care plans place patients with families who provide them with lodging, room, laundry, and personal care. To be eligible for foster care, patients must be ambulatory, free of communicable diseases, able to use toilet facilities without help, and not be in need of skilled nursing care.

Hospice Care.   This service is offered for patients who are in the terminal stages of dementia and can no longer live at home. Hospice environments keep patients as comfortable as possible in their last hours and provide constant counseling and support for families.

Nursing Homes.   Nursing homes are institutions that accept sick patients who are no longer able to live at home. A nursing home falls into one of three categories:

- A *skilled nursing facility* provides intense levels of round-the-clock nursing care by registered nurses, licensed practical nurses, therapists, nurses' aides, and various social services.
- A *health-related facility* provides care for patients who do not require skilled nursing but still need some medical aid and a sheltered environment.
- A *multilevel facility* provides both skilled nursing and regular health-related care. A patient may begin with the former and progress to the latter.

As a rule, foster care is for AD patients in the very early stages of their ailment. Hospice compounds are for those in the last stages of decline. Both have their place, though in most instances caregivers will wish to opt for the third alternative, nursing homes.

All About Nursing Homes

Ownership.   Nursing homes can be owned and run on the following bases:

1. For profit
2. As a voluntary facility owned by a religious or communal organization

3. As a nonprofit public facility owned and operated by government agencies

Private and nonprofit homes often tend to provide better care than government-operated homes, but there are no guarantees in this department, and you should never take anything for granted. It is best to investigate all possibilities before making your decision.

Services. Nursing homes provide three basic services for clients:

1. Medical care: medicines, therapy, and personal health care

2. Domestic services: food, clothing, room, recreation, and atmosphere

3. Personal nursing care: help in eating, toileting, dressing, bathing, and getting around

When considering a particular nursing home, investigate and evaluate all three. Here are some important questions to ask concerning each:

- *Medical care:* What kind of medical care and service are provided by the institution? How many physicians and skilled nurses are on staff? Are a doctor and nurse on the premises at all times or at least on call? Are medical specialists available when needed? How often are patients given checkups, and how thorough are they? What kind of sedation and restraint policy is used on demented persons? How are wandering and sundowning handled? Are dental and rehabilitation services offered? Does the nursing home have access to a pharmacist and an ambulance service? What kinds of medical records are kept, and by whom? What emergency arrangements are offered?

- *Domestic services:* Are the rooms light, airy, pleasantly appointed, and nicely furnished? Are halls, walkways, and bathrooms all clearly marked and provided with nonslip surfaces? Are the access routes well established for wheelchairs or persons using walkers? Are there unseemly odors? Is air conditioning supplied in the summer? Are bathrooms well equipped and safe (check for grab bars, nonslip surfaces, and call buttons). Do the bathrooms afford enough privacy? Are there enough closets, bureaus, and storage areas? Are the mattresses firm? Does the bed have a working call button? What recreations are offered? Do patients seem happy and well treated? Do patients seem to get enough exercise and social stimulation? Is there a snack shop on premises? A library? Television? Access to films? Religious services? Phones? Drinking fountains and bedside water? Is a regular calendar of events offered?

What are the visiting hours? Are children allowed to visit? Do the patients seem generally happy and well looked after?

● *Personal nursing care:* Are the nurses well scrubbed, pleasant, and accommodating? Do they show proper solicitude for the patient? Do they seem confident and competent? Does the nursing staff seem to care? Is the food wholesome and the menu varied? Are patients' specific dietary needs adequately met? Is a nutritionist or dietitian on staff? Are patients kept clean? Are they dressed appropriately and cleanly? Is the linen fresh and relatively new? Are there spots on the sheets or blankets?

Licensing. If a nursing home is licensed, it has met specified medical, personnel, and health standards as established by the laws of the state. It also means that the nursing home agrees to live up to basic standards of care and to provide clients with certain agreed-on services. These standards and services tend to vary somewhat from home to home and state to state, however, so don't assume that just because an institution is licensed (or "accredited," a similar term) it necessarily offers first-rate service. But a licensed nursing home is *probably* better than an unlicensed one.

Finding a Home. Referrals to nursing homes can come from a variety of sources including social workers, clergy, physicians, psychologists, an ADRDA chapter, or the county department of social services. Word of mouth is often a good star to steer your ship by in this area; and it pays to listen to the opinions of other caregivers, especially those who presently have a family member in a nursing home.

Eligibility. Nursing homes, especially the good ones, are frequently filled to capacity. Families must often apply to them in advance with the same intensity and uncertainty as trying to get into a good college or to land a job, though procedures vary from state to state. In New York, for instance, qualifications for a bed in a skilled nursing or health-related facility require that a patient be evaluated via special lengthy screening forms (known as PRI) designed to measure a patient's degree of dependency and incapacity. Other states have their own procedures, but wherever you live, be prepared for paperwork, paperwork, paperwork. Once you have decided on the homes you wish to apply to, your physician or social worker will help guide you through this time-consuming and sometimes frustrating process.

Signing a Contract. Before you sign any contracts or documents with a nursing home, make sure you have read them through thoroughly and that you are aware of all costs involved. Spend several hours going over the details of the agreement, and if you have access to an attorney, have him or her vet it for the fine print. Make sure the following points are mentioned and agreed to in the contract:

- The home guarantees to supply the service of a physician, nurse, and appropriate therapy for the patient (as previously agreed on between you and the institution).
- The home agrees that the monthly rate will cover all board, lodging, laundry and linens, recreation, nursing services, leisure-time programs, hospital gowns, nonprescription medical supplies, special equipment (walkers, syringes, wheelchairs, respirators), and the like. Be sure that all additional costs are specifically listed.
- The contract protects you if you must break the contract or if the patient leaves the institution before the contract time is up.

If the nursing home administration balks at your request to study the document for a few days, take heed: This may be a danger sign. In general, be wary of both glad-hand and strong-arm tactics when it comes time to sign. Go slowly, ask questions, disagree if you feel something is amiss, and don't be talked into anything you don't feel good about.

Paying for It.   Two major concerns here are how much and how you will pay.

Concerning the first question, nursing homes vary enormously in cost; generally speaking, the bigger and brighter the home, the higher the fee. This is not always true, however; sometimes large nursing chains offer better service at lower prices simply because they do such "high-volume" business. At the same time, the small, friendly home around the block may end up providing far more TLC than the biggies, and at cheaper prices—but not inevitably. Before you can be sure of anything, you must shop around, ask for referrals, visit the home in person, talk to other caregivers, and get to know what's what.

Representative prices for nursing facilities are difficult to estimate, as there are so many variations from home to home. Do be prepared to spend $100 to $150 a day (or more) for a health-related facility, $125 to $250 a day (or more) for a skilled nursing facility. When you speak with the personnel at various nursing homes, get a thorough rundown of all prices and services, and be sure that extra costs such as laundry and medical supplies are included in the list.

Now the second question: How will you pay for it? Nursing care is expensive, and unless you have been saving up for it for years (and how many persons save up for a nursing home?), chances are you will need help.

Help, fortunately, comes in several forms, the principals being as follows:

1. *Medicaid*. Medicaid is a joint federal-state program with reimbursement policies that differ from state to state. For example, in New York state, Medicaid covers *all* nursing home costs for patients who can qualify on the basis of *income* (current monetary earnings must be low) and *resources* (property, stocks and bonds, savings, etc., must be sparse). The fine points of state-to-state eligibility qualifications are complex, as might be imagined, and are best sorted out by visiting a local department of social services.

2. *Medicare*. Medicare is a government-sponsored social insurance program designed to cover needy persons over the age of sixty-five. Administered by the Social Security Department through the Health Care Financing Administration, Medicare is a powerful benefactor for acute-care patients remaining in hospitals for limited amounts of time but far less of a boon for long-term nursing home patients. In fact, Medicare will pay for skilled nursing care only if the following conditions have been met:

- The patient has been in a hospital for at least three days in a row before going to the nursing home.
- The patient is admitted to a skilled nursing home within thirty days of discharge from the hospital.
- The nursing home's utilization review committee does not disallow the patient's entry.
- A doctor certifies that the patient needs skilled nursing on a daily basis.
- The patient requires ongoing care for the condition he or she was treated for in the hospital.

It is complicated—and there is more. Medicare will pay only part of certain home care bills, minimal amounts of certain others, and nothing for still others. In most cases, it will pick up the tab for a limited time only, usually no more than one hundred days, often less, and sometimes much less. Though appeals can be lodged at the Medicare office if caregivers believe they have more benefits coming to them, it is generally wise not to depend on Medicare for long-term financial support.

3. *Union and Veteran Benefits*. Veterans and union members may

both qualify for hospitalization aid programs. Inquire locally at your local union office or at a Veterans Administration center.

4. *Life Insurance Policies.* All life insurance policies that belong to the patient should be studied carefully to determine if provision is made for disability waivers that cover the cost of premiums when the patient is disabled. Occasionally in private health insurance plans provision will also be made to pay for some nursing home services.

5. *Life-Care Contracts.* In some states an arrangement can be made between the patient or the patient's family whereby sick persons turn over their entire estate—financial assets, home, investments, etc.—and in return receive lifetime care at a nursing home. This method is prohibited in certain states, allowed in others. Inquiries can be made directly at local nursing homes.

6. *Private Funds.* Persons whose net worth exceeds the Medicaid qualification levels may be forced to finance a nursing home on their own. Private pay rates for nursing homes are not regulated, moreover, and institutions charge what they wish. This arbitrary price policy can be an advantage as well as a disadvantage at times, however, as some homes offer sliding scales and "bargain" rates to families who must rely on private resources. Be aware, what's more, that pay rates for homes will invariably go up, once a year or even more often. In some states you are entitled to a specific number of days' written notice before these raises go into effect.

Further Sources of Help for Caregivers

Telephone Services

Telephone Reassurance.   Some home health care agencies offer a service whereby they telephone homebound caregivers and/or patients once a day, simply to chat and say hello. Since a fee is charged for this service, you might consider going the cheaper route and making a similar arrangement with friends or relatives.

Free Telephone Crisis Intervention Service.   An organization called CONTACT offers free telephone counseling and intervention for just about any type of crisis: family problems, suicide, depression, and more. A church-based organization, CONTACT makes a point of being nondenominational. CONTACT maintains hundreds of offices throughout the country. For their phone number in your area call or write to the national headquarters at the following address:

CONTACT Teleministries USA, Inc.
900 South Arlington Avenue
Harrisburg, PA 17109
717-652-3410

Phone Care Signaling Alarm.   Phone Care is an expensive but potentially lifesaving device for patients and sick caregivers. Installed in the home, it sends out a beeping sound at regular intervals. If the signal is not switched off in a designated amount of time, the Phone Care alarm automatically triggers a prerecorded emergency phone call to several people including the doctor, family members, and friends. The device comes with a pocket unit that allows users to transmit the same message when away from home. Phone Care costs around $800 or more from National Phone Care, Inc., 3109 Hennepin Avenue, Minneapolis, MN 55408.

Phone Help for Patients with Pacemakers.   The International Association of Pacemaker Patients provides an inexpensive service that allows members to test their pacemakers for performance and function from a home phone.

International Association of Pacemaker Patients
610 Equitable Building
100 Peachtree Center
Atlanta, GA 30303

Clergy

One of the jobs that most clergy receive training in is provision of counseling for caretakers of sick persons and for crisis intervention. Inquire at your local church or synagogue for further information.

Public Agencies

Both community and state-sponsored organizations for the elderly can be found in most metropolitan areas. In New York City, for instance, a model agency known as the New York City Alzheimer's Resource Center serves as a comprehensive information, referral, counseling, and public education program to link up AD patients, their families, and professional care providers with appropriate health care services. In 1984, its initial year of operation, the resource center helped more than six thousand persons find needed help and support, and an additional three thousand were reached through public education activities and special seminars. This is typical of the kind of work a good city or state organization can provide. Consult a knowledgeable health care professional or your local phone book for names and addresses.

New York City Alzheimer's Resource Center
  280 Broadway
  New York, NY 10007

Medic-Alert

AD patients and caregivers suffering from serious disorders such as epilepsy or heart problems can register with the Medic-Alert main offices and receive bracelet identification tags. In an emergency, physicians can identify patients and their ailments from these tags and call the Medic-Alert office, open twenty-four hours a day, where further medical information on patients is permanently kept. This service is especially good for demented persons who tend to wander.

Medic-Alert Foundation International
  1000 North Palm Street
  Turlock, CA 95380

Center for Medical Consumers and Health Care Information, Inc.

This group provides caregivers with accurate, up-to-date information on the best health care alternatives for their particular home care situation. The center features a large, free lending library of books on medical subjects, maintains a counseling service, and publishes a newsletter called *Health Facts*.

Center for Medical Consumers and Health Care Information, Inc.
  237 Thompson Street
  New York, NY 10012
  212-674-7105

National Self-Help Clearinghouse

This organization maintains a listing of all the self-help groups in the country and provides referrals for caregivers' specific needs.

National Self-Help Clearinghouse
  Graduate School University Center
  City University of New York
  33 West 42nd Street
  New York, NY 10036

Useful Hotlines

Help is sometimes no farther than your telephone and often no more expensive than the price of a long-distance call. Besides the ADRDA help line, the following can be useful numbers for caretakers:

Alcohol Abuse Hotline 800-ALCOHOL. Operates twenty-four hours a day, seven days a week. Provides counseling for caregivers or demented family members with drinking problems.

Amputation Information Hotline: 718-767-0596. The National Amputation Foundation will advise you and refer you should a demented person need amputation surgery. Operates 10 A.M. to 4 P.M. EST, Monday through Friday.

Grief Hotline: 312-990-0010. An organization called the Compassionate Friends will provide referrals for caregivers who have recently suffered the loss of a loved one. Operates 9 A.M. to 3 P.M. CST, Monday through Friday.

Home Care Hotline: 202-547-7424. The National Association for Home Care provides referrals concerning local medical home care organizations. Operates 9 A.M. to 6 P.M. EST, Monday through Friday.

Pain Control Hotline: 703-368-7357. Operates twenty-four hours a day, seven days a week. This hotline answers all questions pertaining to pain control. (If no one answers, calls will be taken by an answering machine and volunteers will call back collect.)

Suicide Hotline: 213-381-5111. Operates twenty-four hours a day, seven days a week. Provides immediate telephone counseling for persons who are contemplating suicide or for persons with family members at high suicide risk. Also refers callers to suicide prevention clinics.

Surgical Second Opinion Hotline: 800-638-6833. A government-sponsored service that provides information on where to get a second opinion on proposed surgical operations. Operates 8 A.M. to midnight, seven days a week.

Useful Organizations

Administration on Aging
330 Independence Avenue SW
Washington, DC 20201

American Association of Homes for the Aging
1129 20th Street NW (Suite 400)
Washington, DC 20036

American Geriatrics Society
    770 Lexington Avenue (Suite 400)
    New York, NY 10021

Gray Panthers
    2480 16th Street NW (Suite 903)
    Washington, DC 20009

Mental Health Association
    1800 North Kent Street
    Arlington, VA 22209

National Council of Senior Citizens
    925 15th Street NW
    Washington, DC 20005

National Council on Aging
    600 Maryland Avenue SW (West Wing 100)
    Washington, DC 20024

National Institute on Aging
    Public Information Office
    9000 Rockville Pike
    Building 31, Room 5C 35
    Bethesda, MD 20892

Appendix 1

Possible Causes of Alzheimer's Disease

Considering the fact that Alzheimer's dementia has been recognized as a disease only since the 1970s, the speed with which medical understanding of this ailment has increased is remarkable. Though perhaps slowed by lack of finances (private and government funding agencies have not yet fully recognized the epidemiological implications of Alzheimer's), researchers are approaching the problem of the disease's etiology from several directions at once, and to date findings are suggestive of many leads. In fact, some doctors are now concluding that like cancer and heart disease, Alzheimer's disease may result from more than one cause.

What are the strongest contenders so far? The following are all main features on the researchers' agenda:

The Neurotransmitter Lead

We have seen earlier that mental messages are conducted via neural signals, all of which are linked to a cosmically complex series of electrochemical circuits that network their way across the brain. It also happens that the neurons themselves produce substances that aid in this process of intercellular communication. These chemical expediters are known collectively as *neurotransmitters*. They are chemical agents that help nerve signals make the leap across the gap—the synapse—from one neuron to the next. More than a hundred neurotransmitters have been identified in the human nervous system to date; many times this number may yet be discovered.

One of the most important of all neurotransmitters is a chemical known as *acetylcholine*, which, besides carrying nerve signals across intercellular gaps, also helps form salts that reduce blood pressure, triggers peristalsis, and manufactures *choline*, a vitamin B product dear to the hearts of health food aficionados. The chemical workings of this neurotransmitter make up what is called the *cholinergic system*, and it now appears likely that the cholinergic system plays some part in assisting the mechanics of human memory.

Researchers have found, for instance, that if the cholinergic system's production of acetylcholine is blocked by certain drugs such as curare (used by Amazonian Indians to tip their poison darts) or belladonna (once employed by witches to induce trances in their victims), a temporary amnesia ensues that is similar to the kind experienced by Alzheimer's patients.

Interesting also is the fact that researchers have discovered that persons with AD almost invariably show a lack of an enzyme in their systems known as *choline acetyl transferase*, which is required for the production of acetylcholine. AD sufferers also lack *acetylcholinesterase*, which degrades and then removes the acetylcholine after it has performed its task of transmitting a nerve impulse across the synapse.

The discovery of these neurotransmitter deficits has led scientists to believe that the cause of Alzheimer's disease is somehow related to acetylcholine shortages, and the logical conclusion from this supposition is that if more acetylcholine is made available to the starved brain cells of Alzheimer's patients, their memories, as well as several of their other mental functions, could perhaps be restored. Researchers are experimenting with methods for increasing the amounts of acetylcholine in the brain and with techniques for blocking its degradation.

Substances such as *physostigmine*, for instance, are known to inhibit acetylcholinesterase, and thus by a kind of an inverse process to increase the amount of acetylcholine in the brain by decreasing its rate of breakdown. Persons so treated have displayed some improvements in memory skills and in spatial abilities, though problems with physostigmine's toxic side effects have not yet been overcome. Work with another acetylcholinesterase inhibitor, THA, has also shown promising results, and persons so treated have improved in ways described as modest to dramatic. But again, toxicity impedes testing. Nonetheless, work with neurotransmitters seems to be one of the strongest leads that Alzheimer's researchers have come up with so far, and scientists hope to see major breakthroughs in this area within the next several years.

The Toxic Chemical Lead

Aluminum is the most common metal on the earth's crust, so it is not surprising that its traces show up in the neurofibrillary bundles and senile plaques of Alzheimer's sufferers. What *is* surprising is that such relatively large quantities of it appear in AD brains, and in such high concentrations.

This odd observation has caused researchers to speculate on a link between aluminum consumption and dementia. Perhaps we imbibe too much of this metal via cooking utensils, some professionals suggest, or through our food and air. On the island of Guam, where immigrants and natives alike are prey to a form of dementia that produces Alzheimer's-like neurofibrillary tangles and plaques, the deposits of aluminum in the island's bauxite soils are known to be unusually high. Similar observations have been made in other parts of the world where aluminum is heavy in the soil. Scientists in Norway have even hazarded the theory that the real culprit behind AD is the aluminum found in acid rain which, it is known, is mainly responsible for the acidification of lakes and streams around the world.

Yet research has discovered no consistent relationship between exposure to aluminum and lesions in the brains of AD sufferers. It is also known that aluminum levels increase in the brains of aging persons as a matter of course, which may explain why large residues have been observed so frequently among the Alzheimer's population. At one point it was also thought that measuring aluminum concentration in the cerebrospinal fluid could form the basis of a diagnostic test for Alzheimer's, but again, results established no dependable correlations. Nor is there any hard proof that exposure to aluminum in ingested sources such as antacids, cookware, and antiperspirants increases the dementia risk.

Some researchers have thus come to believe that aluminum is not a primary cause of dementia but that since some people develop the disease at age fifty-five and others at eighty, there is the possibility that environmental contaminants such as aluminum hurry the process along. Whatever the case, the high concentrations of aluminum in the brain tissue of demented victims is there for *some* reason, and so research continues.

The Viral Lead

The theory that Alzheimer's disease is contagious and is caused by a virus is based in part on observations made of two rare neurological diseases: kuru and Creutzfeldt-Jakob disease. Kuru (the name means "trembling with fear") is an ailment found only among the eaters of human flesh in the New Guinea highlands. Its symptoms produce lesions somewhat similar to those of Alzheimer's disease, and its victims, curiously enough, are exclusively women and children.

For many years this strange gender and age selection among kuru sufferers mystified researchers. Finally, a field anthropologist living among the kuru-susceptible populations made the telling observation that only women and children of these tribes are allowed to eat the brains of their cooked victims (the men get all the rest), and it took only a minor bit of medical logic to figure out that the disease was transmitted by means of a slow-acting brain virus. This same viral etiology was then found to be common to the slow-acting dementia of Creutzfeldt-Jakob's disease, which also demonstrates characteristics similar to AD (as do certain neurological viral animal diseases such as scrapie and mink encephalopathy), so researchers quite naturally assumed that AD might also be viral in origin.

Unfortunately, assumptions are about as far as the viral hypothesis has been taken. Under laboratory conditions, no clear clinical evidence thus far has been produced to support the virus theory, and there never has been a proven transmission of a supposed Alzheimer's virus in the lab.

At the same time it is a possibility, though admittedly a remote one, that the hypothetical AD virus incorporates itself into the DNA structure and is thus not identifiable via normal methods of observation. Champions of this approach maintain that we need to learn more about the structure of the virus itself before we can reach definitive decisions.

The Genetic Lead

Studies of certain family trees have demonstrated that AD can pass from generation to generation almost like a contagious disease, with as many as 80 percent of family members developing the disorder. Such extremes are rare, however, and most families with an Alzheimer's relative or two are not nearly at such high risk. Still, the question abides: Do persons with a close family member suffering from AD have an increased chance of developing this ailment?

The answer is most likely yes, but with qualifications. Some family pedigrees, it is believed, have a predisposition toward an abnormal marker on one of their chromosomes. Exactly what this marker looks like and precisely where it is located are not yet known. What *is* known is that the predisposition toward this genetic quirk is inherited and that it can be passed down through the family tree. Susceptible family members carry the Alzheimer's gene for life, and for them a family history of the disease is clearly cause for concern.

In practical terms this means that when a person is diagnosed as having AD, that person's first-degree relatives—parents and children—are estimated to have approximately four times the likelihood of developing AD as those without a suspicious family history. These figures have only recently come to light due to the logistic difficulties of studying intergenerational samples, a problem compounded by the ironic fact that since AD does present itself in the later years, carriers of the suspect gene do not always live long enough to express it.

At the same time, some family trees are far more likely to produce Alzheimer's than others. This means that even though a genetic tendency toward dementia exists, this tendency may be slight. Moreover, it would be superstitious to believe that a person who is carrying the supposed Alzheimer's gene is "destined" to develop the ailment. Remember, the odds at work here are genetic *probabilities*, not mathematical certainties, and probabilities, what's more, that are biologically programmed to appear late in life, sometimes so late that before their hour comes, other more common conditions have staked their claim.

Today the genetic lead, though in its incipient stages, remains in the forefront of research, mainly because it is clear that inheritability, along with age itself, is the only key factor we know that in certain cases can be *definitely* linked to the onset of Alzheimer's disease. Research groups are now working toward isolating the factors responsible for genetic transmission and developing early methods for identifying increased risk.

Other Possible Leads

One interesting phenomenon that has perhaps not received the attention it deserves is that brain insults caused by such physical shocks as a fall or a punch to the head can in certain instances increase the likelihood of developing Alzheimer's disease. Persons whose brains have been seriously jarred have sometimes been found to develop a variety of neuritic plaques and neurofibrillary tangles not unlike those observed in

Alzheimer's patients. A conclusion might be hazarded that head trauma in some as yet unrecognized way propagates the factors that lead to AD.

Interesting too is the immunologic approach. This theory posits that for various reasons the body manufactures antibodies that, Frankenstein-like, turn against their creator and destroy the very brain tissue that produced them. This pathological process is not unknown to physicians, who refer to it as an *autoantibody reaction*. Presently it is believed that some autoantibody reactions do, in fact, take place in the brain cells of AD sufferers. But just how and why is uncertain.

Nor is the role of other environmental pollutants besides aluminum thoroughly understood. It may yet turn out that an unrecognized toxin in the environment, perhaps even some substance manufactured within our own bodies, is responsible for producing the lesions that typify AD. It is known, for example, that besides aluminum, silicon levels are elevated in the brains of some Alzheimer's patients and that undue amounts of aluminum silicate (a combination of both chemicals) have been measured in others. What does this mean? Why, moreover, do certain people develop Alzheimer's disease at the relatively young age of fifty-five while others do not show symptoms until they hit their nineties? Could environmental pollutants serve as a catalyst? Possibly. And so the research goes on.

Appendix 2

Picture Flash Cards for Demented Persons

The drawings rendered here by student artist Shawn LeVesque show how it is possible, with a little imagination, to make your own series of helpful flash cards which can then be used to communicate with a nonverbal AD patient. Even after having lost the ability to speak, a demented person often retains the memory of how to respond to visual symbols. The pictures included here are a typical sampling of the situations that arise during the care of a demented person. With a little creative thinking you can come up with your own.

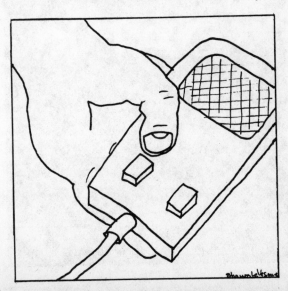

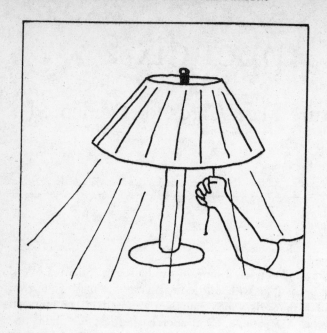

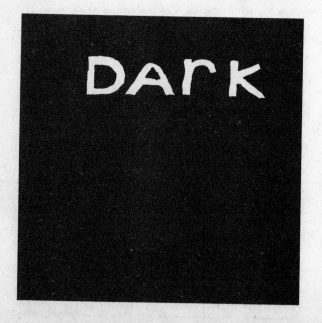

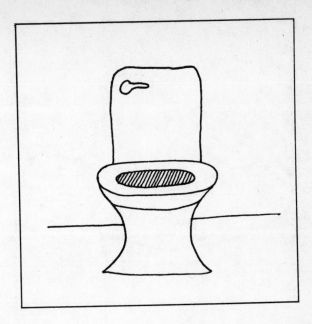

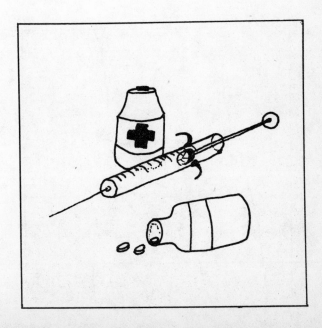

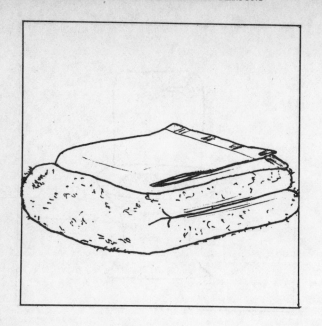

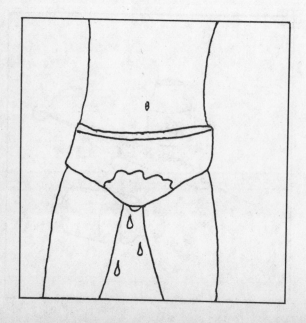

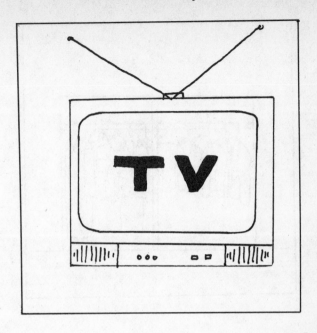

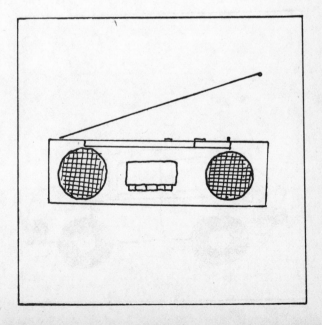

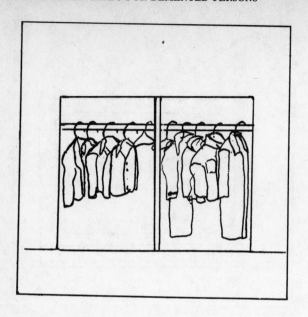

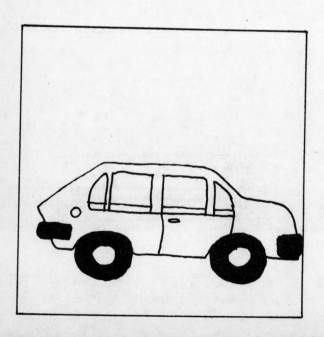

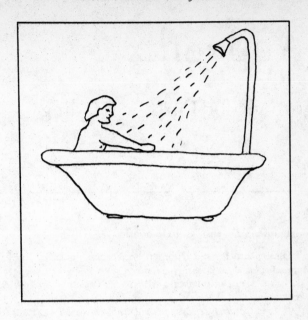

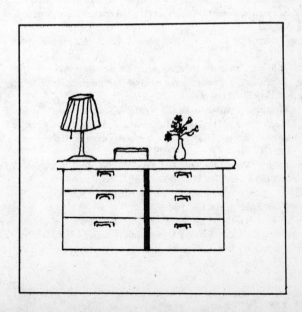

Appendix 3

Suggestions for Further Reading

Alzheimer's Disease and Dementia

Alzheimer's Disease and Related Disorders Association, Inc., 360 North Michigan Avenue, Chicago, IL 60601. *Newsletter.*

Aronson, Miriam K., ed. *Understanding Alzheimer's Disease.* New York: Scribner's, 1988.

Carey, J. R. *How to Create Interiors for the Disabled.* New York: Pantheon Books, 1978.

Chermak, J. *Activities for Patients with Alzheimer's Disease and Related Disorders.* Available from Hillhaven Corporation, 1835 Union Avenue (Suite 100), Memphis, TN 38104.

Cohen, Donna, and Carl Eisdorfer. *The Loss of Self: A Family Resource for the Care of Alzheimer's Disease and Related Disorders.* New York: New American Library, 1986.

Cummings, J., and D. Benson. *Dementia: A Clinical Approach.* Boston: Butterworth, 1983.

Frank, J. *The Silent Epidemic.* Minneapolis: Lerner Publications, 1985.

Gallender, D. *Eating Disorders: Illustrated Techniques for Feeding Disorders.* Springfield, Ill.: Thomas, 1979.

Guthrie, D. *Grandpa Doesn't Know It's Me.* New York: Human Sciences Press, 1986.

Gwyther, Lisa P. *Care of Alzheimer's Patients: A Manual for Nursing Home Staff.* Chicago: American Health Care Association and Alzheimer's Disease and Related Disorders Association, 1985.

Heston, L., and J. White. *Dementia: A Practical Guide to Alzheimer's Disease and Related Illnesses.* New York: Freeman, 1983.

Holland, G. B. *For Sasha, with Love: An Alzheimer's Crusade.* New York: Red Dembner Enterprises Corp., 1985.

Mace, N., and P. Rabins. *The 36-Hour Day: A Family Guide for Persons with Alzheimer's Disease, Related Dementing Illnesses, and Memory Loss in Later Life.* Baltimore: Johns Hopkins University Press, 1981.

Matsuyma, S., and L. Jarvik. *Alzheimer's Disease and Associated Disorders: An International Journal.* Lawrence, Kans.: Western Geriatric Research Institute, n.d.

McDowell, F. H. *Managing the Person with Intellectual Loss at Home.* New York: Burke Rehabilitation Center, 1980.

Middleton, L. *Alzheimer's Family Support Groups: A Manual for Group Facilitators.* Tampa, Fla.: Suncoast Gerontology Center, University of South Florida Medical Center, 1984.

New York City Alzheimer's Resource Center. *Caring: A Family Guide to Managing the Alzheimer's Patient at Home.* 1985.

New York City Alzheimer's Resource Center and New York ADRDA Chapter. *Alzheimer's Disease: Where to Go for Help in New York City.* 1987.

Powell, L. S., and K. Courtice. *Alzheimer's Disease: A Guide for Families.* Reading, Mass.: Addison-Wesley, 1983.

Reisberg, B. *A Guide to Alzheimer's Disease.* New York: Free Press, 1981.

Ringland, E. *Alzheimer's Disease: From Care to Caring.* Rollingbay, Wash.: Healthcare Press, 1984.

Roach, M. *Another Name for Madness.* Boston: Houghton Mifflin, 1985.

Ronch, Judah, *Alzheimer's Disease: A Practical Guide for Those Who Help Others.* New York: Cross & Continuum, 1989.

Seymour, C. *Precipice: Learning to Live with Alzheimer's Disease.* New York: Vantage Press, 1983.

Smith, K. *Aging and Dementia.* Jamaica, N.Y.: Spectrum, 1977.

U.S. Congress, Office of Technology Assessment. *Losing a Million Minds: Confronting the Tragedy of Alzheimer's Disease and Other Dementias.* Washington, D.C.: Government Printing Office, 1987.

Zarit, J., S. Zarit, and N. Orr. *The Hidden Victims of Alzheimer's Disease: Families Under Stress.* New York: New York University Press, 1985.

General and Related Materials

Abreu, B. *Physical Disabilities Manual.* New York: Raven Press, 1981.

American National Red Cross. *American Red Cross Home Nursing Textbook.* New York: Doubleday, 1979.

Barrett, Virginia, and Barry Gurland. *Special Skin Care Problems of the Incontinent Elderly and Their Health Care Providers.* Cincinnati, Ohio: Procter & Gamble, 1987.

Blazer, Dan, and Ilene Siegler. *A Family Approach to Health Care of the Elderly.* Reading, Mass.: Addison-Wesley, 1984.

Bosshardt, J., D. Gibson, and M. Snyder. *Family Survival Handbook: A Guide to the Financial, Legal, and Social Problems of Brain-damaged Adults.* Los Angeles: Family Survival Project for Brain-damaged Adults, 1981.

Bruer, J. *Handbook of Assistive Devices for the Handicapped Aged.* New York: Haworth Press, 1982.

Burnside, Irene. *Working with the Elderly: Group Process and Techniques.* Monterey, Calif.: Wadsworth Health Sciences Division, 1984.

Butler, R. N., and M. Lewis. *Aging and Mental Health*. St. Louis: C. V. Mosby, 1982.

Calder, A., and J. Watt. *I Love You but You Drive Me Crazy: A Guide for Caring Relatives*. Vancouver, Canada: Fforbez, 1981.

Carroll, D. L. *Living with Dying: A Loving Guide for Family and Close Friends*. New York: McGraw-Hill, 1985.

Edwards, H. *What Happened to My Mother?* New York: Harper & Row, 1981.

Flaherty, M. *The Care of the Elderly Person: A Guide for the Licensed Practical Nurse*. St. Louis: C. V. Mosby, 1980.

Gelfand, D., and J. Olsen. *The Aging Network: Programs and Services*. New York: Springer, 1980.

Gold, Margaret. *Guide to Housing Alternatives for Older Citizens*. Mount Vernon, N.Y.: Consumer Reports Books, 1985.

Herr, John, and J. Weakland. *Counseling Elders and Their Families*. New York: Springer, 1979.

Hooker, Susan. *Caring for Elderly People*. London: Routledge & Kegan Paul, 1981.

Hopf, P., and J. Raeber. *Access for the Handicapped*. New York: Van Nostrand Reinhold, 1984.

Jury, D., and M. Jury. *Gramp*. New York: Penguin, 1978.

Karr, K. *What Do I Do: How to Care for, Comfort, and Commune with Your Nursing Home Elder*. New York: Haworth Press, 1985.

Kubler-Ross, E. *On Death and Dying*. New York: Macmillan, 1969.

Nassif, Janet. *The Home Health Care Solution*. New York: Harper & Row, 1985.

Natow, A., and J. Heslin. *Geriatric Nutrition*. New York: Van Nostrand Reinhold, 1984.

Poe, W., and D. Holloway. *Drugs and the Aged*. New York: McGraw-Hill, 1980.

Raschko, B. *Housing Interiors for the Disabled and Elderly*. New York: Van Nostrand Reinhold, 1984.

Safford, F. *Caring for the Mentally Impaired Elderly*. New York: Holt, Rinehart and Winston, 1986.

Shipley, Roger. *The Consumer's Guide to Death, Dying, and Bereavement*. Palm Springs, Calif.: ETC, 1982.

Stern, Jack, and David Carroll. *The Home Medical Handbook: A Patient's Guide to the Most Up-to-Date Treatments, Tests, and Technologies in the Field of Home Care*. New York: Morrow, 1987.

Taira, E., ed. *Physical and Occupational Therapy in Geriatrics*. New York: Haworth Press, 1984.

U.S. Department of Health and Human Services. *Guide to Health Insurance for People with Medicare*, Publication No. HCFA-02110. Available from U.S. Department of Health and Human Services, Health Care Financing Administration, Baltimore, MD 21207.

Villaverde, M., and C. MacMillan. *Ailments of Aging: From Symptom to Treatment*. New York: Van Nostrand Reinhold, 1984.

Weinstein, E. A. *Denial of Illness*. Springfield, Ill.: Thomas, 1955.

Weiss, J. *Expressive Therapy with Elders and the Disabled*. New York: Haworth Press, 1984.

Ziegenfuss, J. *Patients' Rights and Professional Practice*. New York: Van Nostrand Reinhold, 1984.

Index